EXPRESS MAKEUP

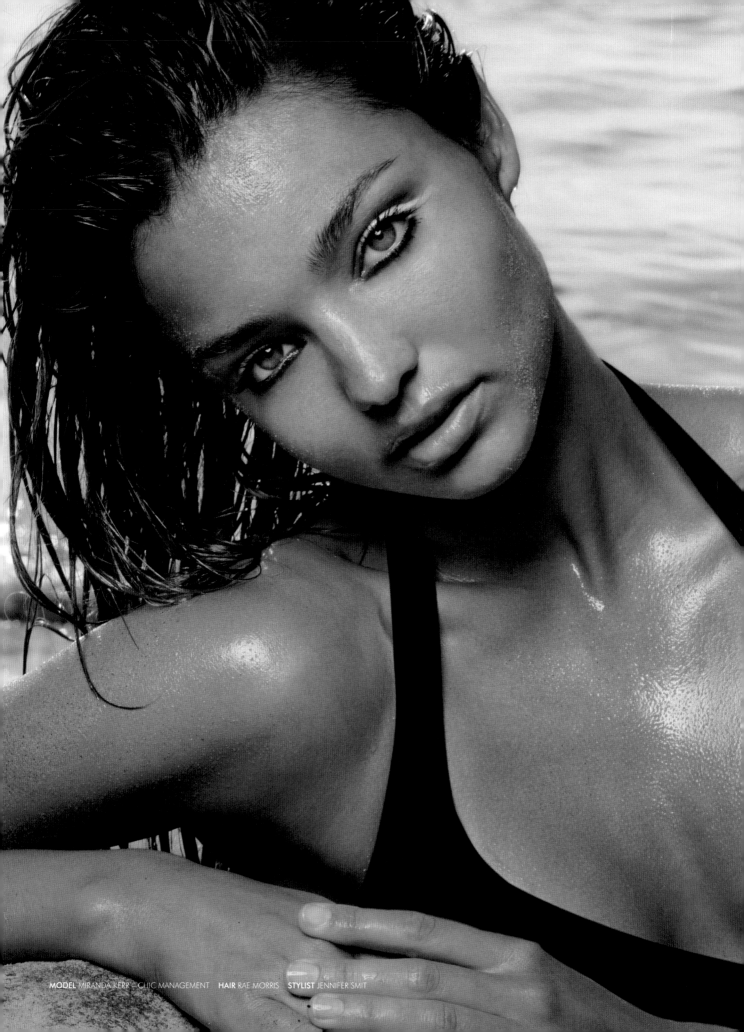

RAE MORRIS

EXPRESS MAKEUP

PHOTOGRAPHY BY STEVEN CHEE

ARENA
ALLEN&UNWIN

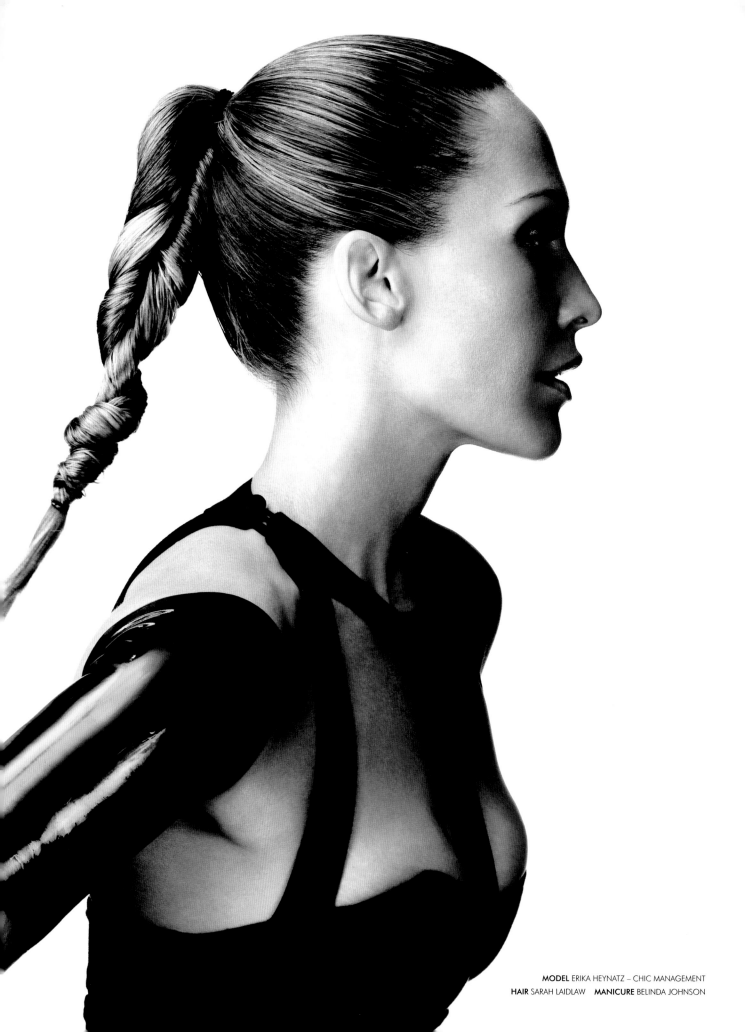

Foreword

For any performer, hair and make-up artists are crucial. They can make you feel like a million dollars on days when you can hardly bear to look in the mirror, and they have the ability and expertise to transform you completely. They are fundamental to what we do, and the best ones can make all the difference in the world.

I first had the pleasure of working with Rae on a video clip I did five years ago, and immediately understood why she's one of the most respected makeup artists in the industry. She is extremely creative, loves a challenge, and her understanding of the female face is incredible! She always makes you feel beautiful and you always know you're in safe hands with her. Rae has an enthusiasm and passion that has seen her work with many international artists, from Kelly Rowland to Pink. She has also won numerous awards and done the makeup for magazines as varied as *Vogue* and *Rolling Stone*.

So clearly Rae is technically brilliant, but I believe that what really sets her apart as a makeup artist is her huge passion and hunger for what she does as well as her uncanny knack of 'getting' who you are and knowing exactly what will make you look and feel your very best. I love Rae's *Express Makeup* book because it is exquisite to look at and allows you to recreate Rae's magic effortlessly. Some of the profits from the book go to UNICEF, who work for children's rights, their survival, development and protection, across the world. That means you can feel beautiful on both the inside and outside when you buy this book, which I, for one, highly recommend.

Natalie Bassingthwaighte

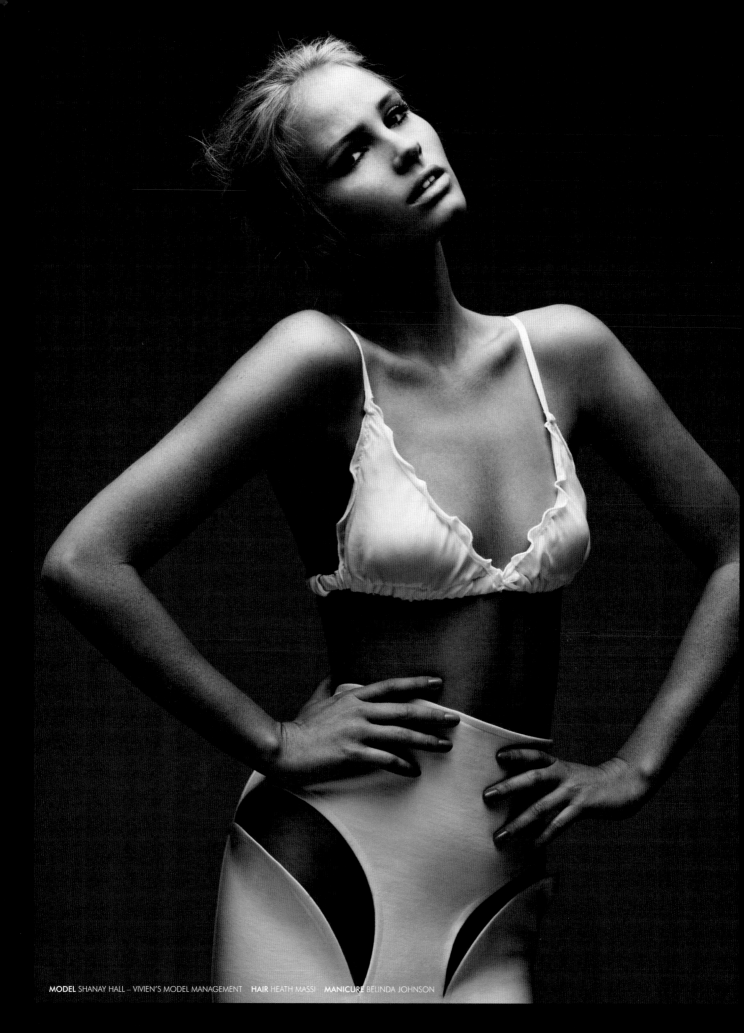

MODEL SHANAY HALL – VIVIEN'S MODEL MANAGEMENT   **HAIR** HEATH MASSI   **MANICURE** BELINDA JOHNSON

CONTENTS

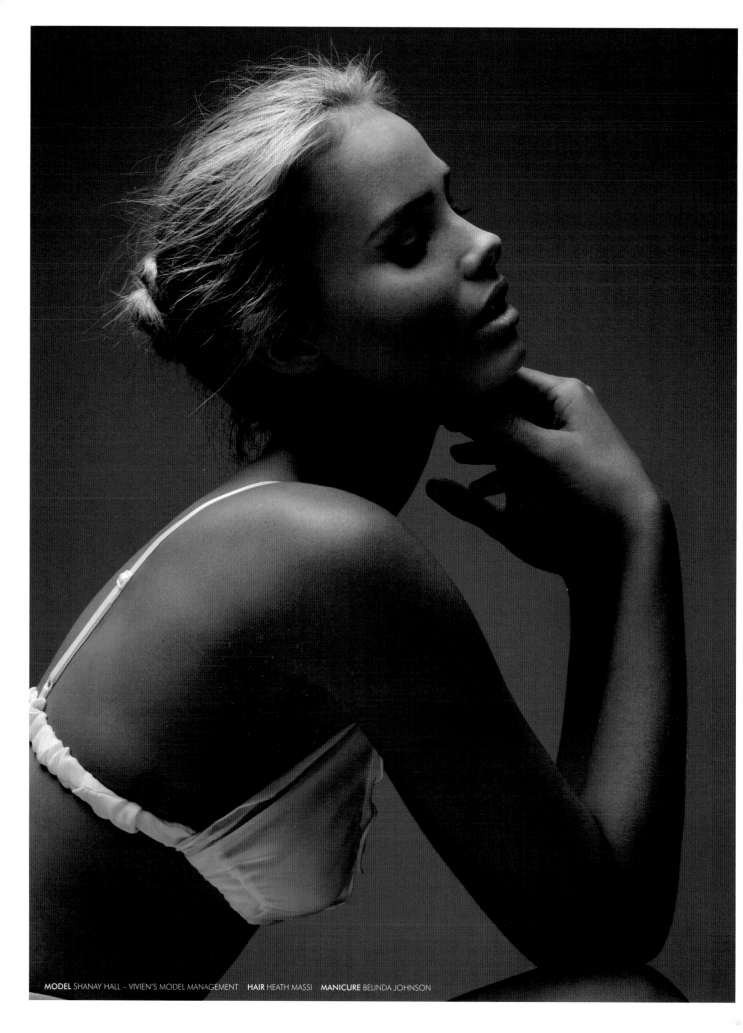

Introduction

For those of you who haven't read my first book, *Makeup: The Ultimate Guide* (2008), my career as an international makeup artist began while I was working as a hairdresser at a beauty pageant in 1993. I'd never done makeup before then because, to be honest, I never really thought I'd be that good at it. I can't draw, and to this day I have to get illustrators to refine my face charts. So the idea of becoming a makeup artist was completely foreign to me.

The only way I can explain what happened that day is fate. It so happened that one of the guest judges at this beauty pageant was Naomi Campbell. At one point during her preparation, Naomi and her makeup artist had a tiff, and he stormed out. As she glared around the room, her eyes met mine and she said, 'Fix my lips.'

Just as I was nervously applying gloss to Naomi's lips, the paparazzi burst through the door. All I remember were blinding white flashes, but the next day photos of me applying Naomi Campbell's lip gloss were plastered everywhere. And before I knew it, I was being booked as a makeup artist. Five minutes of Naomi's life completely changed mine, so I'd like to thank her for the dummy spit that began my career.

A big part of my job involves working backstage at fashion shows, where everything has to be done quickly. The tricks I've learnt over the years are the inspiration for this book, which is about creating beautiful makeup looks fast. You can use it if you have fifteen minutes to spare or just five. There are express fixes for when you're rushing out after work as well as easy-to-achieve looks for a fabulous evening event when you don't have much time.

This book is also for the women who are put off by the thought of how long it takes them to do their makeup. I guarantee that even a piece of sticky tape can help make it perfect in less than a minute, while the simplest reshaping of your brow can completely transform your eye shape. And my number one tip? If time is of the essence, always do your eyes first because you can apply your foundation and lipstick as you're literally racing out the door.

Every woman can do her own makeup by following my expert tips and looks, all of which have beautiful step-by-step photographs and clear instructions. Remember to follow the order given in each step-by-step, as it will increase your speed. There are also some great tips for women over 40.

It's all about your brushes. You can do more with minimal product and an incredible brush range than with cotton buds and drawers of makeup. After using every makeup brush on the planet, I know the good ones are hard to come by, so I've put together the ultimate brush range. Every brush I've chosen is the best of its type; I have done all the research and testing for you. You can purchase them direct from my website: www.raemorris.com.

To me, this book is about more than makeup—it's about how you feel about yourself, which determines how you face the world. I hope this book helps make you look and feel *fabulous*.

1

EXPRESS MAKEUP KIT

WHETHER YOU'RE DOING A KILLER
LOOK OR A QUICK FIX, HERE'S MY
RUNDOWN ON THE BASIC TOOLS
FOR YOUR EXPRESS MAKEUP KIT.

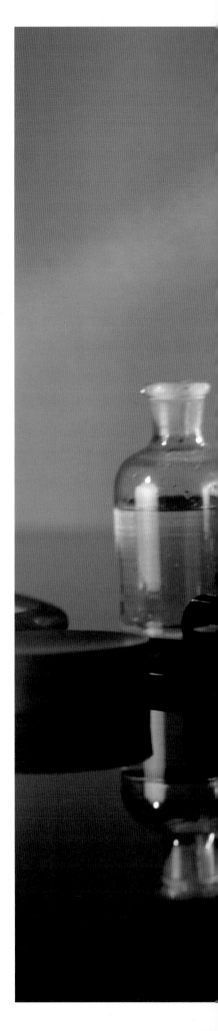

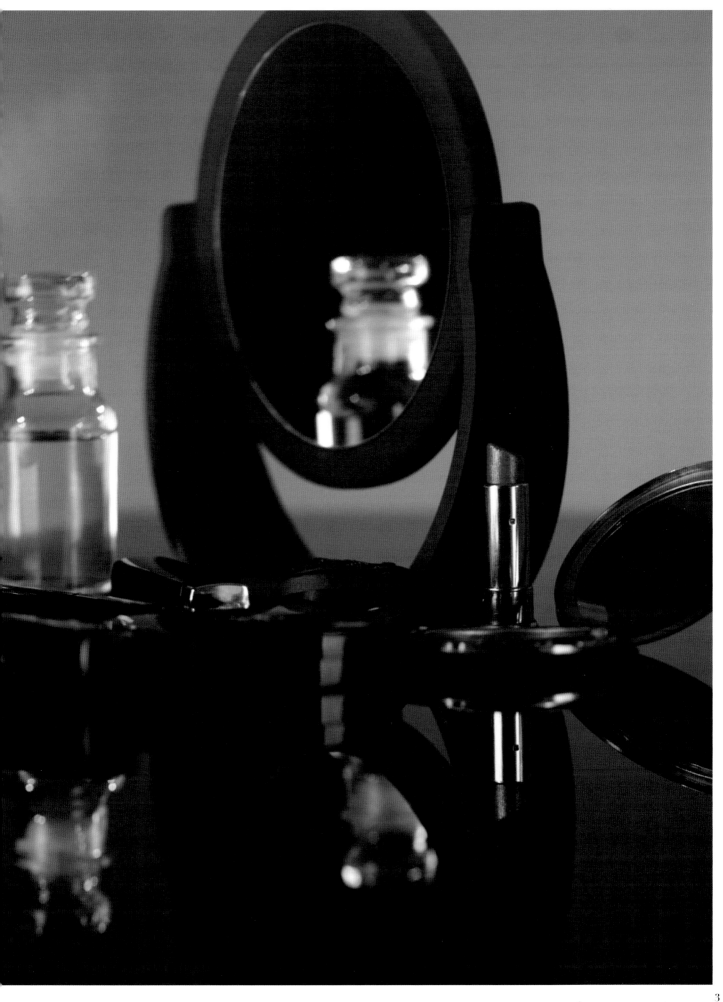

I'm going to get straight to the point. Just a few essential tools will revolutionise the way you do your makeup as well as reduce the time it takes. Fingers and cotton buds just won't cut it.

If you prep your skin properly, and follow all the steps and tips outlined in this section, I guarantee your makeup will last twice as long. And you'll save time, as touch-ups will be minimised.

Here's a rundown on what you need, but don't despair—you may well own half these already. You'll find these tools in every professional makeup kit. Make sure you regularly check the shelf life of these items, as it's important to dispose of anything that's out of date.

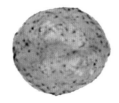

FACE & BODY SCRUB

To make a fabulous facial/body scrub—the best and cheapest you can ever imagine—mix together equal parts of bicarbonate of soda and any good-quality water-based cleanser from your pharmacy. For your face, use about half a teaspoon of each; for your whole body, use a handful of each. Combine these with a bit of warm water, and don't be afraid to get between your eyebrows and over your lips. This mix is recommended by many dermatologists as the gentlest and most non-reactant exfoliant. However, if you're reluctant, try it on your hand first.

Exfoliate your skin no more than once a week. Do not exfoliate at all if you are having chemical peels or using any products that contain Retin As, AHAs or BHAs. If you're undergoing treatment with a dermatologist, check with him or her first.

BABY WIPES

Always use non-alcoholic, non-perfumed baby wipes, as they contain fewer chemicals, thereby reducing the risk of skin reactions.

PRIMER & MOISTURISER

Makeup primer and moisturiser are essentially the same thing, except that a primer has more silicon, which is great for levelling out an uneven skin texture.

My golden rule is to use either primer *or* moisturiser under your foundation, as foundation needs to go into the skin and look like skin. Using more than one product underneath foundation makes it separate and look patchy, and it just doesn't last as long. So don't use both, and make sure that the one you choose contains a sunscreen.

It's important to ensure that your foundation, concealer, primer, sunscreen and moisturiser are all either oil-based or water-based. For example, if you're using an oil-based primer or moisturiser, then make sure your foundation is also oil-based. Similarly, if you're using a water-based primer or moisturiser, you need to use a water-based foundation.

Water-based products generally have the word 'aqua' in their list of ingredients, while oil-based products will list some sort of oil as their first ingredient. The oil-based products tend to slide off your face, so I prefer water-based products, which last longer.

BRUSHES

You don't have to spend lots of money on makeup brushes. I've searched the world for top-quality, inexpensive brushes to use every day for my ultimate brush roll—all the brushes you need, selected by me, in one roll. Go to www.raemorris.com and buy them online. To test a brush you already have, stand it on its tip on the back of your hand—if the bristles collapse, replace the brush.

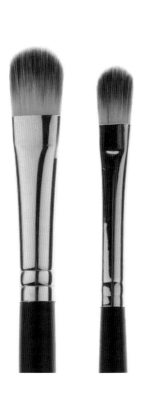

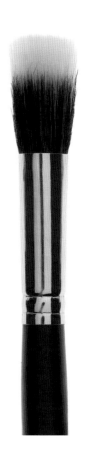

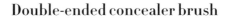

Double-ended concealer brush

This two-in-one concealer brush is fantastic for contouring on the cheekbone and concealing blemishes under the eye. It's quite firm, allowing you to cover problem areas accurately.

Fibre-optic foundation brush

This fantastic brush makes any foundation look flawless. Use it with all types of foundation. The porous white-tipped bristles absorb a lot of liquid, so only dip about a quarter of the brush in your foundation or, alternatively, apply it with your fingertips and just use the brush to blend.

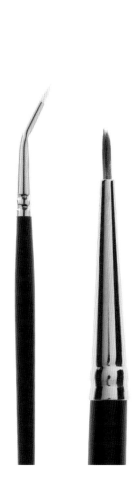

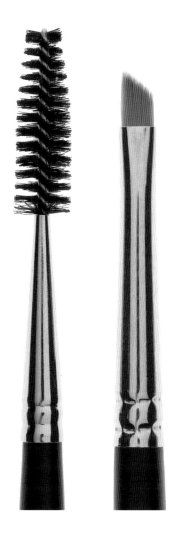

Eyeliner brushes

These two eyeliner brushes are the only ones you'll ever need—the fine eyeliner brush on the right and the hooked version on the left. The latter is great for applying eyeliner to the inner corners of your eyes. Its bent shape means you can get right into the inner eye crease without your fingers getting in the way. And if you have one tiny blemish, either brush can do double duty as a mini concealer brush.

Combined mascara wand/angle brush

This is my number one brush—I couldn't do makeup without it. Use the wand end to comb your eyebrows and remove clumps of mascara. Use the angled end to apply eyeliner, get eye product into the lash line and define your brows. If your lipstick is beginning to bleed, dip the angled end in foundation, and retrace the outline of your lips to redefine them.

The best way to clean your brushes is with brush cleaner, which is available from professional makeup stores. With just one dip, you can sterilise all your brushes to hospital standards, and they dry within seconds. I clean my brushes about twenty times a day, and it doesn't affect the quality. One 5-litre bottle of brush cleaner will last you for at least five years. The alternative is to wash your brushes in hot, soapy water no less than once a week, then rinse well.

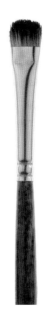

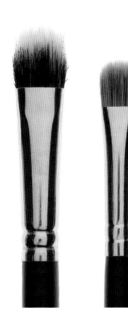

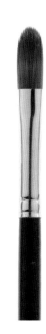

Mini square blending brush

This brush is essential for blending eyeliner or eye shadow around the eyelash line. Its small size helps you keep your eye shadow perfectly in place.

Eye shadow blending brushes

Yes, ladies, having only one blending brush won't cut it; I own about fifty, so you should invest in at least three. Choose each brush depending on the size of the area you wish to cover— the larger the area, the larger the brush, and vice versa.

Lip brush

If you use a firm synthetic lip brush that is slightly longer and stronger than the standard lip brush, you'll avoid those unwanted stray brush hairs that ruin your lip line. Also, a synthetic brush doesn't absorb as much product, so more ends up on your lips.

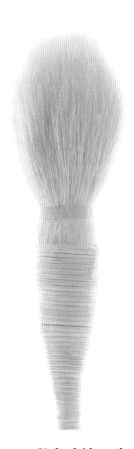

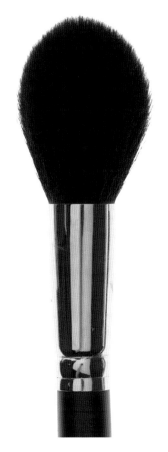

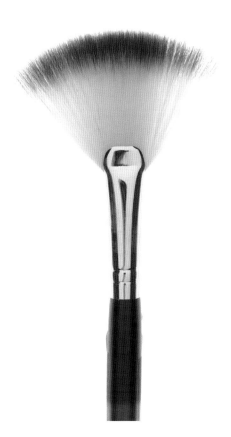

Kabuki brush

I could not do my job without this little miracle brush. It's like a ball of cotton wool and does just about everything, from powdering to applying blush, bronzer and highlighter. You can use it to contour and blend eye shadow, all without leaving awful brush marks. Buy at least two.

Powder brush

I mainly use a powder brush to apply shimmer to the body or, rarely, as a substitute for a kabuki brush. Use it to powder or bronze, but be careful when using it to apply blush because if it's too big your blush may go from your forehead to your jawline. And if it's flat on the end, it will leave edges that are hard to blend.

Fan brush

The fan brush is great for highlighting your cheekbones and various parts of your body, such as your collar bone. It also helps remove messy fallout after you've applied eye shadow.

FOUNDATION

You need two to three shades of foundation so you can match the colour of your foundation to your skin tone all year round. There are so many different types that deciding what to buy can be overwhelming. Here's a list of what's available.

- *Liquid-based: for all skin types, but first check whether it's water- or oil-based. Sheer to medium coverage.*
- *Grease-based: for mature skin, and dry or scarred skin. Medium to heavy coverage.*
- *Oil-based: for dry skin, and to achieve an anti-shine effect.*
- *Water-based: for sheer coverage on all skin types. My favourite!*
- *Powder-based mineral foundation: for a velvety texture on all skin types.*

Foundations also offer several different types of coverage: for stunning skin with no blemishes, go for invisible; for subtle blemishes or slight pigmentation, choose sheer; for heavily blemished skin, choose medium and high.

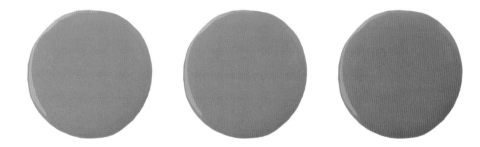

BLUSH

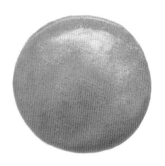

There are two types of blush—cream and powder. Only use powder blush on top of powder foundation and/or face powder, or cream blush on top of liquid or cream foundation.

BLOTTING PAPERS & POWDERS

If you want to matte down your skin with powder without creating a cakey effect, blot your skin with non-powdered blotting papers first. Or simply use them whenever your skin looks too shiny.

Face powders come in two basic forms—compressed and translucent.

HIGHLIGHTERS

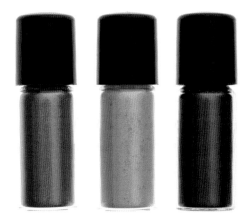

These come in two types—cream or powder—and shades range between a shimmery cream and a deep golden bronze. To find the exact shade to suit you, and also how to apply it, see 'Highlight', pages 68–75.

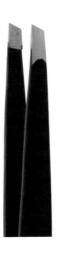

TWEEZERS

Not much explanation required here. Always use tweezers on an angle so you don't stab yourself. And make sure they're easy to grip. When you need to resharpen them, just use a metal nail file. To clean tweezers, wipe them with a cotton bud dipped in antiseptic.

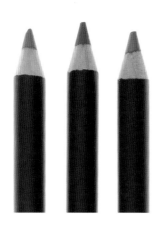

BROW PENCILS

Besides the perfect foundation, your eyebrows are the most important feature on your face, so it's worth buying good brow pencils.

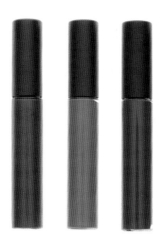

BROW MASCARAS

I've used this amazing little secret throughout the book. Brow mascaras are normally used to temporarily conceal grey regrowth in eyebrows and on hairlines. They are rare and hard to find but great for temporarily lightening or darkening, covering grey and for matching the colour of your brows to your natural hair colour.

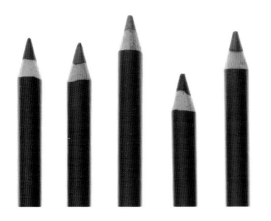

KOHL PENCILS

These are fabulous for both the inner rims and around the eyes. They have a lot more pigment and a lot more intensity than generic eye pencils. And because they're waxy, they feel comfortable, especially on the inner rims of your eyes. Buy pencil eyeliners in each of these essential colours—black, grey, deep brown and creamy white.

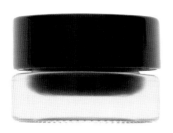

GEL EYELINERS

You only get one chance to nail eyeliner, and I always recommend a gel eyeliner over a liquid one, as liquid eyeliner tends to crack. Gel eyeliners are easy to use and don't dry as fast as liquid eyeliner, so you have more time to blend. And when they're dry, they're waterproof. Always apply gel eyeliners quickly with a sharp-angled brush.

If you've been wearing eye shadow for a while and it has fallen onto the top of your eyelashes, use liquid eyeliner to darken them.

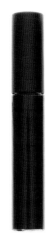

LIQUID EYELINERS

Liquid eyeliners leave no room for mistakes. The only time I use them is to intensify blackness around the eyelash line—for example, after I've done a smoky eye.

EYE SHADOWS

Stay away from cream eye shadows, as they crease in seconds. When buying eye shadows, look for the richest, most intense pigments you can find. Test this by wiping eye shadow with your clean fingertip once. If that's your desired colour, buy it, but if you have to apply it several times to achieve the intensity of colour you want, give it a miss. You can always soften down an intense colour with translucent powder.

For your express makeup kit you need at least three eye shadow colours—a neutral colour, one that intensifies your eye colour and one that highlights it. To find your perfect eye shadow colours—the ones that will complement and highlight your eye colour—see the eye colour charts on pages 49–57.

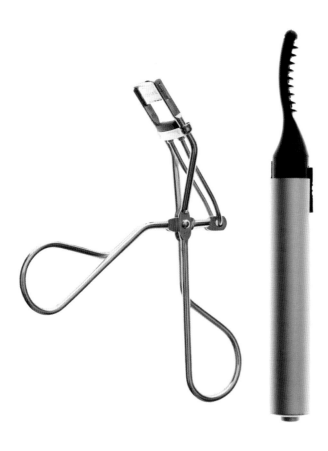

EYELASH CURLERS

Don't spend hours doing fabulous
smoky eyes then leave your lashes
looking like straight fence posts!
If your lashes don't curl naturally,
use a manual eyelash curler before
applying mascara. You can also buy
a mini lash curler (left) for those odd
hairs you just can't reach.

If you're terrified of eyelash curlers,
buy a heated one (right). You can use
both these before and after mascara.
The gentle warmth of the heated
curler is comforting, whereas the
manual type can pinch your eyelids
if it's not used correctly.

MASCARA

I only use black mascara on eyelashes, as brown or grey shades make your
lashes look dirty and unfinished. Once you use the 'comb' mascara you'll never
use a wand again. Note: waterproof mascaras do not break your lashes—it's the
way you remove your mascara—so always have waterproof remover on hand!

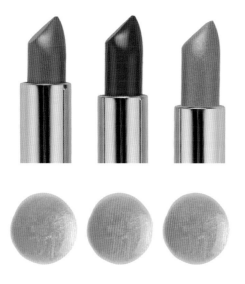

LIPSTICK & LIP GLOSS

If you're confused about what colour lipstick suits you, go for mahogany (think of your natural lip colour, but intensified). It suits everybody, and it's the only shade in the colour wheel that is both 'cool' and 'warm'. So, whatever your age, skin tone or hair colour, it's perfect. And there's a bonus—mahogany lipstick makes your teeth look whiter.

Other lip essentials are your signature lipstick colour, the colour that suits you perfectly and makes you look and feel great; a clear lip gloss and a tinted one; and a gold or shimmery gloss highlighter. I only use lip pencil if I want a matte effect, and I always colour in the whole lip.

If your lipstick suddenly smells or tastes different, chances are it's gone off. Throw it out immediately.

SHOPPING LIST

Skin

- [ ] Skin scrub (bicarbonate of soda + water-based moisturiser)
- [ ] Moisturiser
- [ ] Primer
- [ ] Anti-shine primer
- [ ] Foundation
- [ ] Concealer
- [ ] Powder (if required)
- [ ] Highlighters
- [ ] Luminiser (if required)
- [ ] Bronzer
- [ ] Blush
- [ ] Contour cream
- [ ] Sunscreen

Eyes

- [ ] Tweezers
- [ ] Brow pencils
- [ ] Brow mascaras
- [ ] Kohl pencils (black, grey, deep brown and creamy white)
- [ ] Gel or liquid eyeliner
- [ ] Eye shadows/pigments (at least three different colours)
- [ ] Mascara
- [ ] Eyelash curlers
- [ ] False lashes
- [ ] Eyelash applicator
- [ ] Latex
- [ ] Sticky tape (for eyeliner)
- [ ] Eye drops

Lips

- [ ] Lipstick
- [ ] Lip gloss
- [ ] Lip pencil
- [ ] Lip balm

Hands

- [ ] Hand cream (also great for cracked heels)
- [ ] Cuticle oil

Makeup brushes

- [ ] Brush cleaner
- [ ] Double-ended concealer brush
- [ ] Fibre-optic foundation brush
- [ ] Eyeliner brushes
- [ ] Combined mascara wand/angle brush
- [ ] Mini square blending brush
- [ ] Eye shadow blending brushes
- [ ] Lip brush
- [ ] Kabuki brush
- [ ] Powder brush
- [ ] Fan brush
- [ ] Disposable mascara wands (or clean the one you're about to throw out)

Other essentials

- [ ] Non-perfumed, non-alcoholic baby wipes
- [ ] Blotting papers—non-powdered
- [ ] Makeup remover
- [ ] Waterproof makeup remover
- [ ] Tissues
- [ ] Hair clips
- [ ] Cotton buds
- [ ] Manicure scissors
- [ ] Cotton pads
- [ ] Hand mirror

Express fixes

Use your express makeup kit to touch up your makeup—fast. Here are some quick tips.

Skin

If your skin is too shiny, use non-powdered blotting papers (see page 11). They'll de-shine your skin in seconds and work better than powder.

Tone down flushed skin with an anti-red primer. These are available at your cosmetic or pharmacy counter.

In hot weather, use a grease-based foundation, as it's water-resistant. However, if your foundation is dripping, cool your face down first. Drink some cold water, wet a towel and throw it in the freezer for a minute, then wrap it around your neck to cool down your body. Alternatively, wrap a few ice cubes in a fresh cleaning cloth—preferably not one you've just used to wipe down the kitchen bench—and tie it around your neck. This is how we cool down actors and models on set during a heatwave. Another tip is to keep a cheap battery-operated face fan in your bag. It's safe, light and compact. I've used one on Hugh Jackman many times.

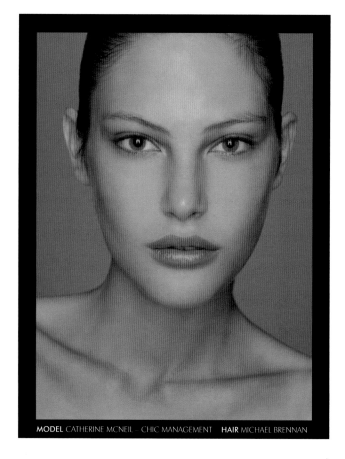

MODEL CATHERINE MCNEIL CHIC MANAGEMENT **HAIR** MICHAEL BRENNAN

Eyes

If you're always in a rush, consider keeping your eyebrows and lashes tinted to your desired colour, and invest in lash extensions so you don't need to apply mascara. They look incredibly natural and can last up to six weeks. Waterproof mascara also helps.

When your mascara runs, squirt some foundation on the end of a cotton bud and use it as an eraser.

If your curled lashes are starting to straighten out like fence posts, warm up a heated eyelash curler and redo.

Before using a cotton bud to touch up around your eyes, especially the inner rims, wet it with eye drops. You'll not only soothe your eyes but also reduce the risk of leaving behind any fibres.

Lips

Apply lip balm heavily to dry lips before you even start your makeup, then let it soak in. By the time you apply lipstick, you'll have luscious, soft lips that will make your lipstick easier to apply. It'll last longer too. I love using lip balm on cuticles, cracked heels and crusty elbows.

Bleeding lipstick? If more of your lipstick is heading south than is actually on your lips, wipe the whole lot off with a baby wipe and start again. But the real trick is to buy the most intense colours and only apply lipstick once—the less product on your lips, the less it will run.

If your lip shape is responding to gravity, don't draw attention to it by applying a bright shade of lipstick. Try this simple test. Apply your brightest lipstick, then look in the mirror, squinting your eyes until your vision is blurred. If your lip shape is youthful and full, go for your life! If it looks aged and lined, choose a nude lip colour, which will give the illusion of fuller lips by making your lip borders less defined. If you want to add more colour to your face, you'll be better off adding more blush and mascara, and brightening your hair colour.

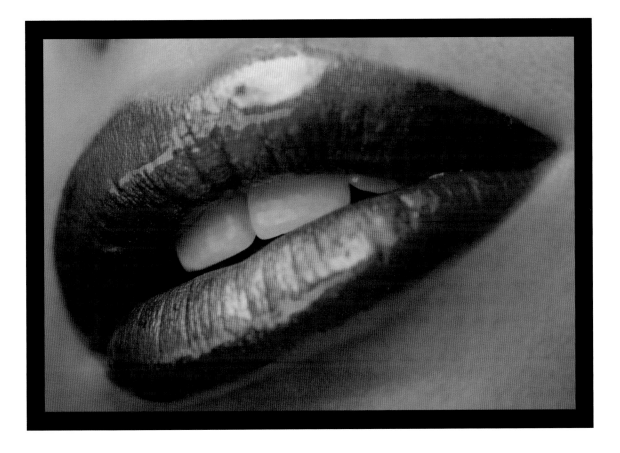

Hands

Resist the temptation to wear red nail polish if you have red hands—it has exactly the same effect as adding a red lipstick to red skin! Instead, wear skin-toned matte polishes.

Apply foundation to the backs of your hands to even out the skin tone and make them look years younger, then clean any foundation from your palms with a baby wipe.

For chipped, unmanicured nails, buy a nail buffer and use it to shine your natural nails. Believe me, you'll have the same shine as if you've used a clear nail polish.

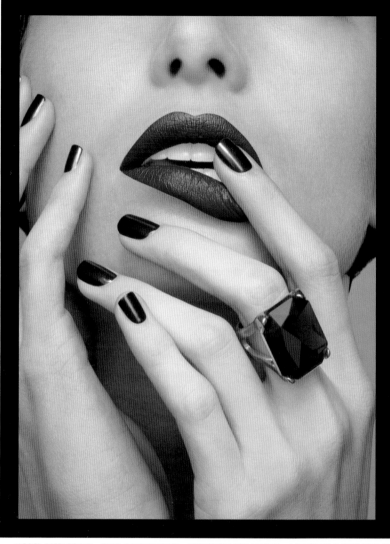

MODEL CASSI COLVIN – **CHIC MANAGEMENT**   **STYLIST** RICHARD MILVAIN   **MANICURE** MANDY LEVANAH

Hair

For greasy hair, use dry shampoo, which looks like deodorant in a can. It transforms greasy hair in seconds.

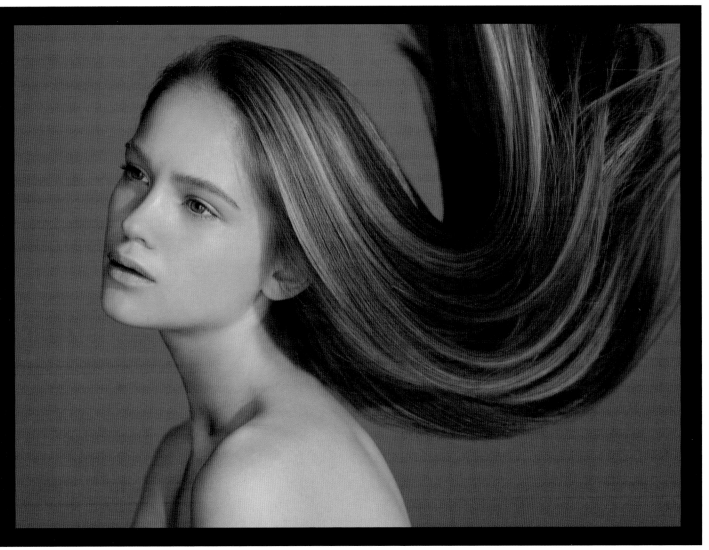

MODEL ROSIE TUPPER – VIVA LONDON (LONDON) & DNA (NEW YORK)   **HAIR** HEATH MASSI

After 5

If you're getting dressed up for a special night out, then you're probably adding bling to your ears, décolletage and hands. In other words, you're highlighting potential problem areas, which, depending on your age, may make you look years older. If your earlobes have become saggy from wearing heavy earrings, wear something a bit discreet and delicate. And if you can't resist wearing a plunging neckline but your décolletage concerns you, blend your makeup down to your dress rather than stop at your jawline. Use mineral foundation to cover this area, as it has a flawless finish as well as the best staying power; it is also less likely to appear on your clothes. Alternatively, simply wear a scarf.

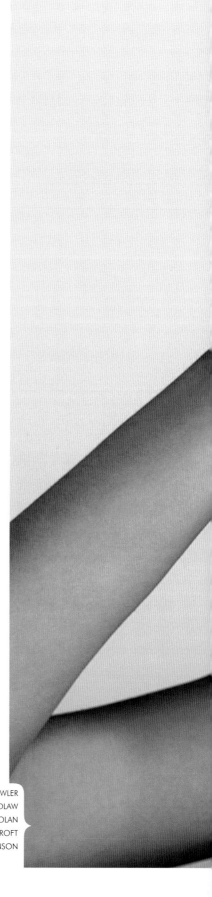

2 EYE & SKIN PREP

FOLLOW THESE STEPS AND
YOU'LL COMPLETE YOUR
MAKEUP IN HALF THE TIME.

MODEL GEORGIA FOWLER
HAIR SARAH LAIDLAW
STYLING GEOFFREY NOLAN
ART DIRECTION BENJAMIN CROFT
MANICURE BELINDA JOHNSON

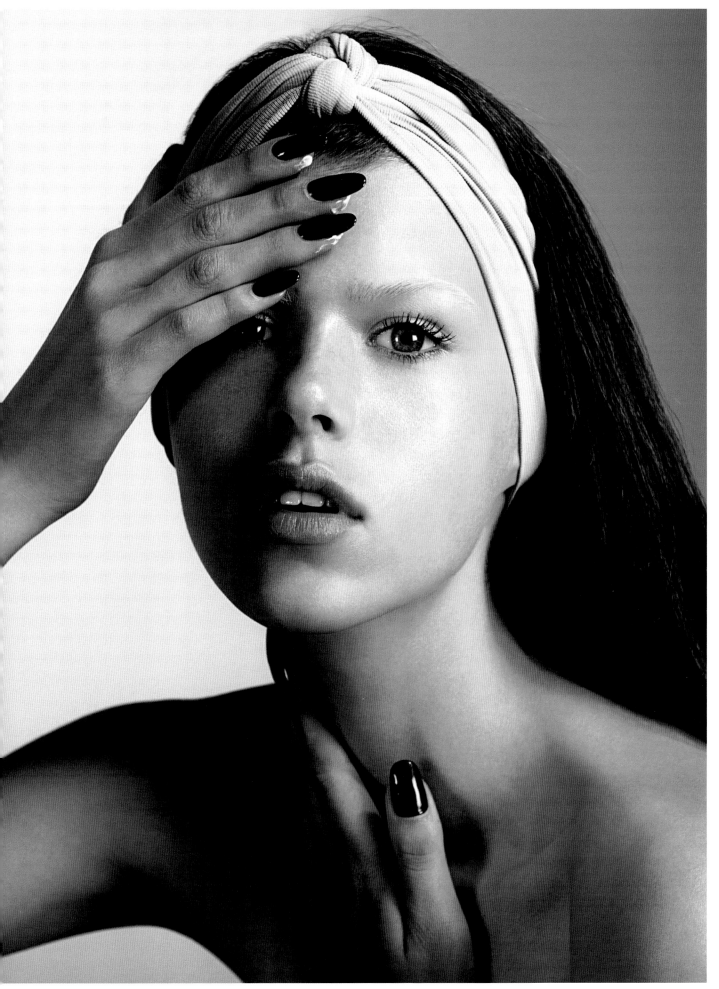

There are two ways to prep your skin. The first way is obvious—prep your whole face by cleansing, moisturising and the weekly scrub. But there is an 'express' prep you can do when you've had makeup on all day and you just need to freshen up.

You don't have to start all over again and do the works. You can simply refresh your whole look by prepping your eyes. Not only will you apply makeup faster, but also your eye shadow will look more vibrant and last longer. The eyelids are one of the oiliest parts of the face, so when I do makeup, whether the model is 15 or 50, I remove all the oil from the eyelids first. The eye makeup will then last for 6 to 8 hours without me having to retouch.

Why eye shadow doesn't last

The biggest killers of eye makeup are natural oils and any form of moisturiser around the eyes. As you read this, rub your index finger across your eyelid to feel the oil. I guarantee it's there! It's impossible to blend eye shadow on a very oily lid surface. Generally your eyelids are as oily, if not oilier, than your T-zone, and this is why eye shadow creases. (Your T-zone includes your centre forehead, the corners of your nostrils, the tip of your nose, your top lip and the middle of your chin.)

Follow these steps to start your makeup from scratch after work or before a night out but, if you don't have time to take everything off and start again, just refresh your eyes.

CLEANSE

If you're nowhere near running water, use a non-alcoholic, non-perfumed baby wipe on your face and eyelids—a great tip if you're at the office and about to go out. Not only will it remove all the oil, these wipes leave no residue, so you can apply makeup straight on top. (All the others leave behind an oily residue that must be rinsed off; also, they can irritate your skin.)

PRIME / MOISTURISE

Here's the golden rule—only use one product beneath your foundation. Foundation needs to disappear into the skin, not sit on top (see 'Primer & moisturiser', page 5).

APPLY FOUNDATION & CONCEALER

Don't moisten your eyelids. Instead, put a light amount of foundation on your eyelids and/or concealer under your eyes. If you tend to have dark patches under your eyes, you may find your foundation is sufficient. But if it isn't, apply some concealer as well, and let your eye makeup begin.

The other reason why you shouldn't moisten your eyelids is that all foundations contain some form of moisture anyway, so you'll be doubling up in an area that just doesn't need it.

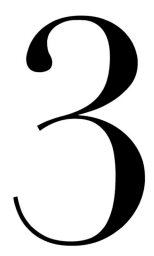

3 <u>FOUNDATION</u>

LEARN HOW TO CREATE LUMINOUS,
FLAWLESS SKIN THAT MATCHES YOUR
SKIN TONE PERFECTLY.

MODEL GEORGIA FOWLER
HAIR SARAH LAIDLAW
STYLING GEOFFREY NOLAN
ART DIRECTION BENJAMIN CROFT
MANICURE BELINDA JOHNSON

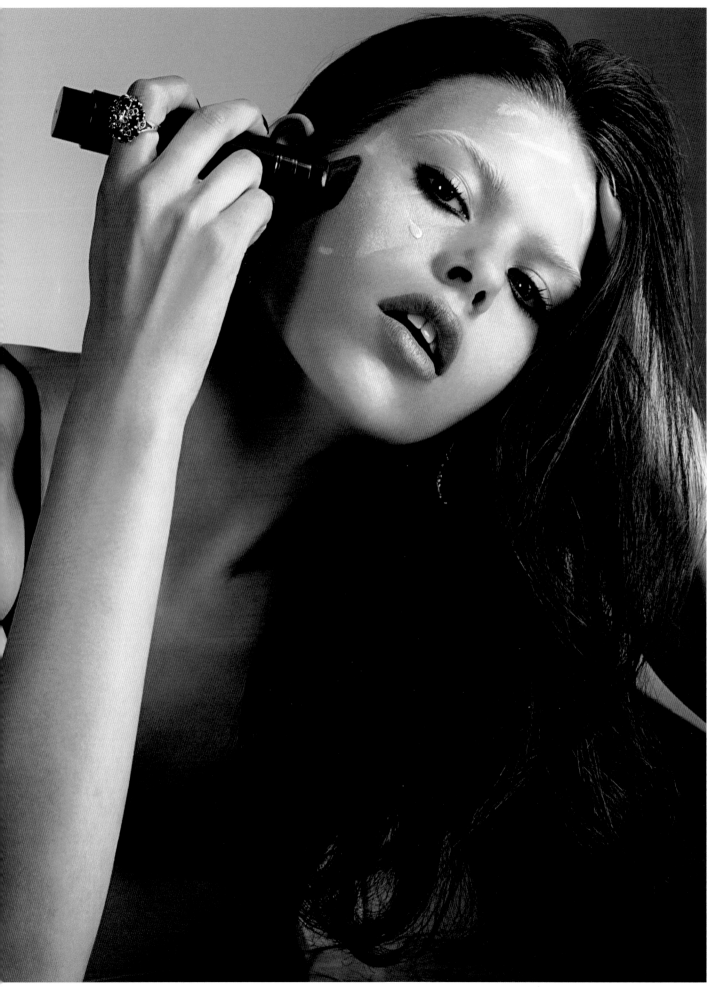

I can't believe how many foundations are available in the market today. Since I wrote *Makeup: The Ultimate Guide* (2008), a million more claims—including lightening, anti-ageing, plumping and luminising—have been made for various foundations. I just wish there were a greater colour selection available, rather than a huge number of ranges.

I want to simplify what seems like a very complex product, and make it very straightforward and easy for you to purchase foundation next time you hit the makeup counter.

This is not a skincare book—a whole topic on its own—so I don't have time to go into skin reactions or sensitivities. To find out more about skincare, just hit the internet, type in 'skincare' and check out the thousands of sites at your fingertips.

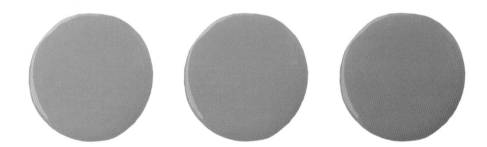

Your skin type

Before you decide on a foundation, put yourself in one of these two categories.

NORMAL / OILY / BLEMISHED

Before you apply any foundation, first prep your skin (see pages 24–5). As your skin already has a generous supply of oil, a water-based foundation is best. Only use water-based moisturiser or primer in areas that are not excessively oily. Never go for a matte foundation, as it's too different to your natural texture. Sure, your skin, especially your T-zone, may grease up during the day, but you can easily remove the sheen by using non-powdered blotting papers as often as you like. (The colour of a powdered blotting paper may not match your skin colour.) This also keeps your skin creamy, so you can constantly reapply concealer or foundation as required. Remember, once you powder, you can never just refresh your foundation—you'll have to take everything off and start all over again.

If you really want to achieve a velvety or matte skin, always blot before you powder, and remember that halfway through the day you may need to remove your whole foundation and start again. You can apply a good foundation in less than three minutes and leave your eye makeup intact.

NORMAL / DRY

If you have this skin type, you may feel as though you've drawn the short straw; so many people talk about how lucky they are to have oily skin, as it keeps their skin looking youthful. But guess what? Normal to dry skin is a dream for long-lasting foundation. Just exfoliate once a week with the magical bicarb and moisturiser mix I recommend in 'Face & body scrub', page 4.

Always use a primer or moisturiser, and go for creamier, even, oil-based foundation. Your skin will drink it up like a sponge. And if you want a matte finish, go for it. Even if your skin feels dry, you may tend to get a bit of shine around the nose or forehead. Simply blot your T-zone with non-powdered blotting papers before you apply any powder. However, I must say I rarely powder dry skin.

Skin texture

When you choose foundation, your number one decision is based on one factor only, and that is the skin 'texture' you want. (To find your perfect foundation, see 'Finding your perfect colour match', page 36.)

Listed opposite are all the textures I create nearly every day. If you choose the wrong texture, it can make you look ten years older. To give you a visual of how powerful the texture of your base is, think of the most popular eye makeup—the classic liquid black eyeliner. Now think of how different the same eyeliner looks on 1940s screen actresses (matte foundation) versus Angelina Jolie (soft, creamy skin). Then compare them to Jennifer Lopez (dewy skin) to appreciate how the texture affects the look of your makeup.

Look at the list of foundation textures opposite and decide on the end result you want. And try experimenting—you might like to mix an eye look with one of the following foundations.

Only use tinted sunscreens on blemish-free skin, as they don't provide good coverage.

Foundation textures

Here's a list of the different foundation textures, all of which are included in this book.

- *Sheer:* *Minimal coverage and an invisible finish.*

- *Soft dewy/creamy:* *Light to medium coverage.*

- *Glowing/luminous:* *Creamy, with extra shine.*

- *Velvety finish:* *Bare skin or foundation powdered with very sheer translucent powder.*

- *Heavy coverage:* *Creamy, dewy finish (great for covering scars and blemishes).*

- *Heavy coverage:* *Matte finish.*

Remember, your foundation type can change the look of your whole makeup, so choose the one that suits you best.

Powder

My number one rule with foundation is to *never powder* your base just to make your makeup last longer. Yes, powder your skin if you want the finished look to be velvety/less shiny or matte, but never powder your base. Here's why.

Let's say, for example, that your non-powdered foundation lasts perfectly on your skin for three hours before it starts to slightly separate and deteriorate. As a result, you decide to pick up some powder and apply it, hoping for an all-day lasting effect (which is impossible). When you do this, you change your desired youthful dewy skin to powdered matte skin and, believe me, no one is going to look at you and wonder, 'Wow, I wonder how long your makeup's lasted?' They're just thinking how caked and flat your skin looks.

Yes, powdering your foundation will make it last a little longer, but not as long as you think (it usually adds only an extra hour or two), and it also creates all sorts of problems with reapplication. The second you powder your skin, you can never go back and reapply your cream concealer or liquid foundation to touch up—you can only reapply more powder. And we all know how that starts to look after a few attempts.

You may not want to hear this, but some of the most fabulous makeups just don't last. For example, incredibly glossy red lips need to be constantly touched up; dewy, creamy foundations applied to oily skin need to be blotted and de-shined; and glossy eyelids crease in a matter of minutes. That's why, as a makeup artist, I very rarely do a celebrity then take the rest of the day off. I'm there hour after hour, touching up.

Also remember that some of the textures you want to achieve just don't last as long as others. In my opinion, some of the foundations that claim to last for three days can create the most hideous, ageing, caked-on, nanna-looking effect you can ever imagine. Wouldn't you rather look more youthful, and occasionally reapply, than look as if you're wearing a granny mask, just because you're too lazy to touch up occasionally?

Anti-shine primer

If you're a shiner, I have a solution for you—buy a packet of either non-powdered blotting papers (see page 11) or some anti-shine primer, an incredible cream that makes excess oil evaporate. Your skin will look instantly matte. This primer, once only available to professional makeup artists, is now filtering through to the mainstream. Use it only on oily skin or your T-zone, for obvious reasons. Apply it with either a sponge or a foundation brush.

If you're now excited about this product, and can't find it in the department stores, call a professional makeup supplier in your area and ask for an anti-shine primer. They may even be happy to provide a demonstration.

Anti-shine primer is mainly used on men who have greasy facial skin and don't want to wear even a hint of makeup. It's also amazing on bald-headed men whose heads shine like light bulbs.

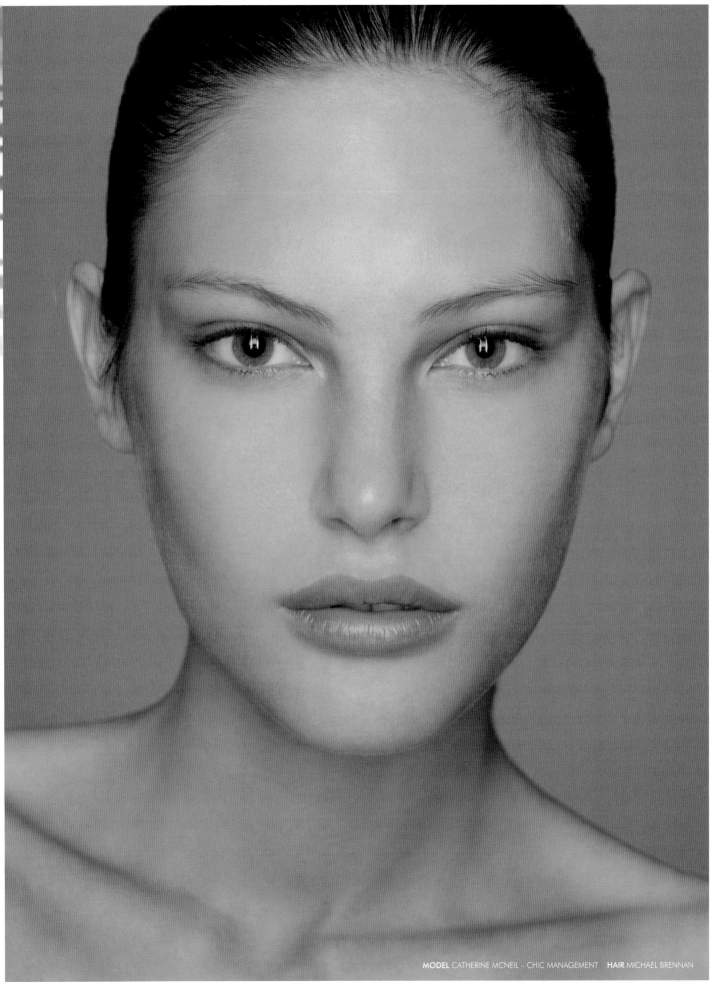

33

Mineral foundations

I hope that by the time you're reading this book, women aren't still over-whelmed and confused by this incredible makeup craze. Actually, it's more than a craze because I predict we're moving into a makeup generation in which all makeup—including lip gloss, blush and possibly even mascara—will become mineral. I love mineral foundations, by the way, as they're great on sensitive skins and most of them have sunscreens.

I don't really understand why this fabulous invention confuses so many women—the only difference is that it's applied with a special application brush. Only choose the powdered version if you desire a velvety matte finish. For a dewy, creamy effect, choose the liquid one.

Powdered mineral foundations come with a brush because they have a powdered texture, and need to be polished into the skin, not lightly dusted over it. Women who love the mineral revolution tend to go heavy on the oily moisturisers prior to application, but by the time mineral foundation hits moisturised oily skin, it sticks like glue.

So only lightly moisturise your skin before you apply mineral foundation. I'd even recommend that you let your moisturiser settle for a few minutes until it's completely absorbed before applying your mineral foundation.

Luminisers

One of the most fabulous tricks of the trade, these pots of golden creamy sheen come in at least three shades, suitable for pale, medium and black skins. Giving your skin an incredible glow is so easy to achieve. Simply add a couple of drops to your foundation and *voilà*—your skin is now luminised. Think Miranda Kerr, J-Lo or Anne Hathaway.

Highlighters

When you only want to shimmer up certain areas of your face, see my easy, step-by-step instructions in 'Highlight', pages 72–4. For instance, if your skin is heavily blemished or scarred, only shimmer certain features rather than give your face an all-over glow.

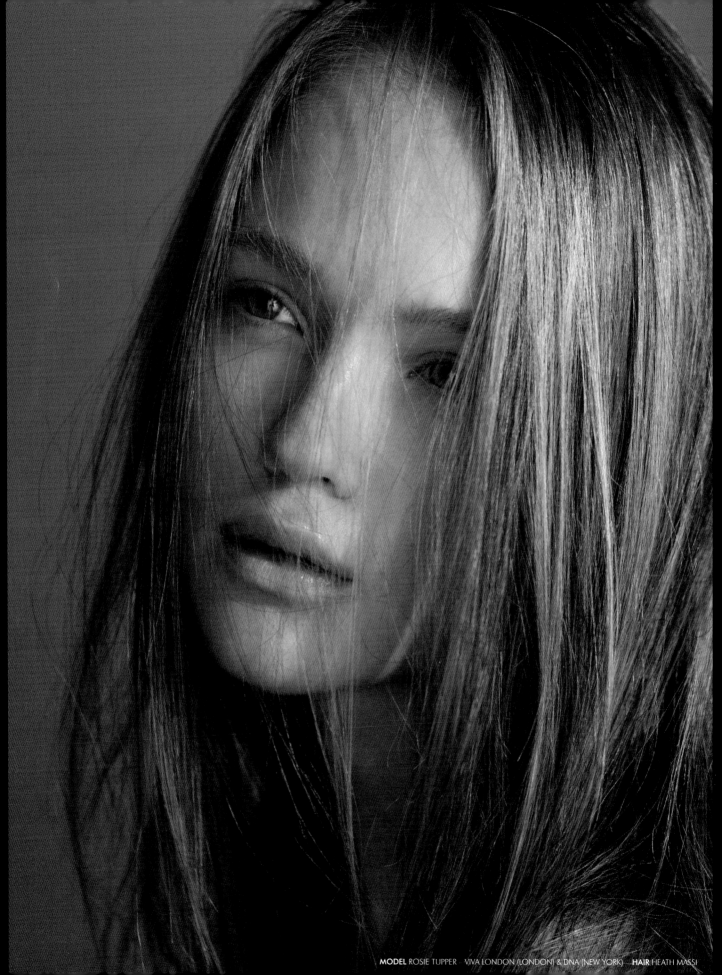

Finding your perfect colour match

There's one basic rule for choosing the right colour of foundation—match your foundation to the colour of your collarbone/décolletage (chest area). It's essential that your face and body are the same colour. If your skin tans, changing tone from summer to winter, always change your foundation to match! I believe every woman should own a minimum of two shades.

With this in mind, try the following exercise. Put on a singlet top and apply the foundation you currently use. Turn side on to the mirror and put your chin onto your shoulder. Your forehead should be the same colour as your chin, shoulder, arm, knee, even right down to your ankle. Think of two extreme skin tones—say, Anne Hathaway's versus Beyoncé's. Their foreheads match their chests, their shoulders, their knees, their elbows.

Never match your foundation to your jawline, as your neck area is one of the palest parts of your body.

Applying foundation

Throughout this book, you'll constantly see the foundation brush I've used to apply different foundations (see 'Brushes', page 6). I *never* use a sponge. (And it's years since I've seen another professional makeup artist use one.) A sponge may seem like a cheap alternative, but it's expensive in the long run because more foundation is absorbed by the sponge than by your skin. And if you don't wash it after *every* use, it will be full of bacteria.

I always use either my hands or a brush. My favourite brush for applying foundation is the fibre-optic brush (see page 6). If you want to use your hands, apply foundation in the same way you would moisturiser. It's that easy.

Natural daylight is best for applying makeup; never leave the house without checking your makeup in the most natural light. And if you're doing your makeup at night, make sure your globe is the type that replicates natural daylight. The best place for checking makeup is in the rear-view mirror of a car, because it reflects so much natural light back onto your face. It's also a great way to pick up those few stray lip or eyebrow hairs.

Installing soft glowing makeup lights in your bathroom may make you feel like a supermodel, even without makeup, but step outside and you could well be horrified by how many mistakes you've made.

Concealing blemishes

When I was growing up, all we had for skin breakouts were toothpaste and highly alcoholic toners. These days, dermatologists and cosmetic doctors can do incredible things. So, if blemishes are ruining your life, consult a dermatologist or a highly trained cosmetic doctor.

I've witnessed the miraculous things these experts can achieve. I've seen acne disappear, scars literally removed and blemishes fade overnight. And although this book is about speedy makeup application, not skin care, one type of cream worth finding out about is Retin A, a wonder cream for skin. It has incredible anti-ageing effects, clearing skins in a way I've never seen before. It may not suit everybody, but it's definitely worth asking your dermatologist.

Choosing the right concealer

Always buy highly densely pigmented concealers, as you can always blend them down. Here's a trick for testing a concealer at the makeup counter: use a red felt pen to draw a tiny red circle on the back of your hand, then go to a department store. Try different concealers until you find one that can cover that red spot completely and still leave your skin looking like skin.

Applying concealer

The following rule applies to all makeup: any makeup that is lighter than your skin's natural shade will highlight and raise indentations, while any makeup that is darker than your skin's natural shade will have the opposite effect— it will flatten.

If you're covering a scar or deep, dark circles under your eyes, or anything that sits below the skin's surface, such as a hole or dint, choose a concealer that's one to two shades paler than your foundation.

But if, on the other hand, you're concealing a blemish or a mole or a raised imperfection (in other words, something that's above the skin's surface), you need to choose a concealer that is the exact shade of your foundation, maybe even half a shade darker, so that it will flatten and minimise. You concealer-crazy fans may not realise that using a light concealer on a raised blemish will actually highlight it!

Bronzing

Bronzer is the most misused makeup product on the market.

The aim of bronzing is to make you look as if you've just come back from a wonderful holiday on an exotic island, not like you're coming down with glandular fever or jaundice. Yet so many women get this wrong.

Bronzer, especially in the powdered blush forms, is meant for skin that already has a slight natural tan—in other words, to enhance what you already have. Using it on pale skin does not make you look more tanned—it makes you look as if you're wearing two big orange doughnuts on your face.

A true tan has various tones, because your skin doesn't tan evenly, with the nose and forehead generally tanning up to two shades darker than the rest of your face. Yet some women apply powdered bronzer evenly (and often heavily) all over their face, because they think it gives them more colour. Well, it does—a muddy brown one. And why on earth would you want to make your face darker than your body?

The perfect way to look more tanned is to either luminise your skin (see 'Highlight', page 66), or make your foundation shade a little darker. Again, do this only if it matches your body colour. If you have medium to dark skin, you can bronze away to give yourself that Beyoncé glow. On the other hand, if you have pale skin, you need to darken your body colour if you want to tan your face. The best tip for 'twilighters' is to create a healthy look by just giving your lips and cheeks a brighter shade.

So here's how to bronze (see also pages 96–7 for the step-by-step technique).

1 In a perfect world go to a salon and get a spray tan. And yes, have your face tanned as well (or if you're an expert, do it yourself at home).

2 If you have pale skin, don't use bronzer straight on your skin. However, if you must, mix a little with your blush colour. Women with pale skin should stick to peachy pinkish blushes, not brown, because the latter is too dark and heavy, making their skin look dirty.

3 Know your bronzing limit—choose a bronzer that is only a few shades darker than your natural skin tone. For example, if you have light skin, choose subtle shades (such as the colour of bamboo); for medium skin, go for terracotta; and for dark skin, choose deep tan shades.

4 If you're using a powdered bronzer, avoid patchiness by first lightly dusting your face with translucent powder. This will help with blending. However, if you wish to use a cream bronzer, just apply it directly onto cleansed skin or straight on top of your liquid or cream-based foundation.

I haven't included instructions on full body bronzing, as this book is about express makeup and bronzing takes time! However, if you want to know more about bronzing, see the tips below, and also the 'Bronzing' chapter in *Makeup: The Ultimate Guide* (2008).

Bronzing tips

- *For a light, even finish, always apply bronzer with a clean brush (the kabuki is my favourite).*
- *Be careful when applying bronzer around your jawline. If you overdo it, you'll look as if you have a 5 o'clock shadow.*
- *Don't use shimmery bronzers if you have excessively oily skin or fine lines. Instead, opt for a matte version.*
- *Make sure you blend bronzers down to your neck area — don't stop at your jawline. Your neck is always paler than your face because your chin shades it from the sun.*
- *Before you apply bronzer, add a hint of rose-coloured blush to your cheeks to give a natural healthy look.*
- *Check the shelf life of the product — they generally last 6 to 12 months.*

4
FALSE EYELASHES

TRANSFORM YOUR LOOK
WITH THE BEST ACCESSORY
YOU'LL EVER OWN.

MODEL GEORGIA FOWLER
HAIR SARAH LAIDLAW
STYLING GEOFFREY NOLAN
ART DIRECTION BENJAMIN CROFT
MANICURE BELINDA JOHNSON

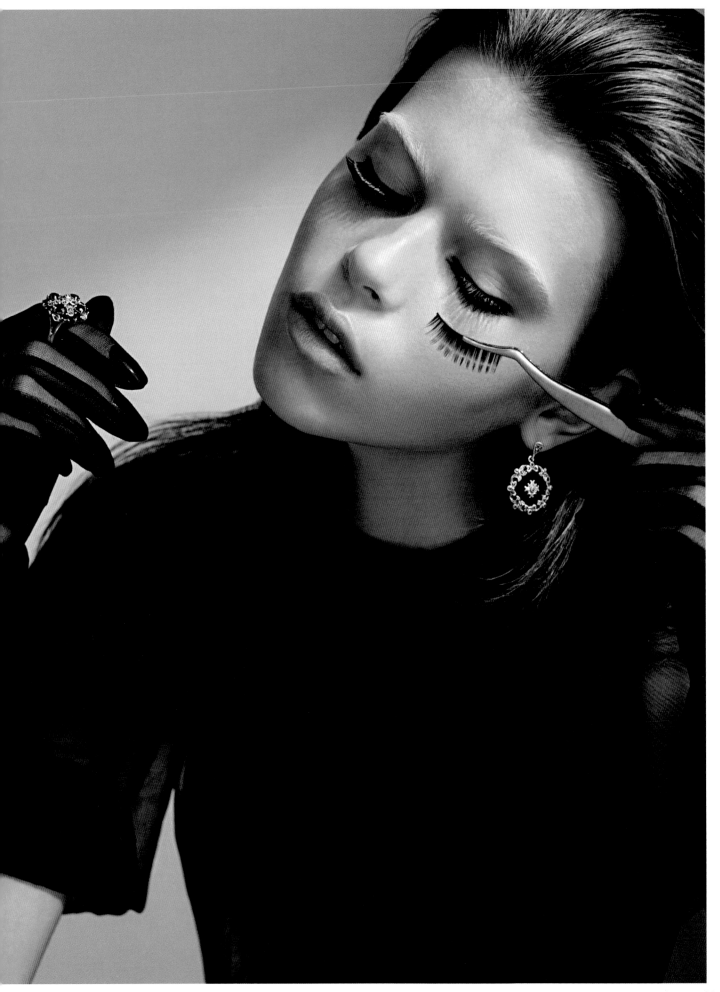

Please don't be overwhelmed by the title of this chapter. For one, false eyelashes should never look 'false' and, two, with the correct tools it takes only a few minutes to put them on. Nothing can change or enhance an eye as quickly as a false lash. If you're still overwhelmed, remember that you'll never have runny mascara again. Great for weddings and tear-jerker movies!

As this is an express makeup book, I'm only going to talk about false eyelashes that are quick and easy to apply (these might be hard to find, so look up my faves on www.raemorris.com—these are the best available and the easiest to apply). If you're buying them elsewhere, remember to check that they're an *exact* fit, because they completely change both your eye shape and the overall look of your makeup.

Always apply lashes with latex. Most lashes come with a small complimentary tube, but it's great if you can track down one that's made with duo latex, which can be found in every makeup artist's kit. And make sure the latex is water-proof: otherwise, if you cry, and the latex is not waterproof, they'll fall off.

I've also discovered a magic tool, known as an eyelash applicator (also available on my website). I don't know how I ever applied lashes without them.

Before a special night out, it's worth practising applying false eyelashes. Always check the base of the lash, which will be either clear or black. This is the seam to which all the lashes are sown. If the seam is black, you will get an eyeliner effect on your eyelids. If it's clear, they will look more natural, blending in with your own lashes without giving that eyeliner effect.

As you browse through the following steps, you'll be able to see the difference between clear- and black-seamed lashes. You'll also see how powerful false eyelashes can be. All I've changed are the model's lashes, not the makeup, which is very basic. I've just curled her natural lashes and applied a fine, soft wash of mascara. To remove lashes, just use warm water on a cotton pad. If you hold the cotton bud over your eye for about two minutes, the latex should easily fall away. In most cases you can reuse false lashes.

Don't apply false lashes the whole length of your lash line, as they'll drag down your eye. Always move them in a millimetre or two from the outer edge.

NATURAL

In this shot our model is wearing only a little mascara on her natural lashes, no other eye makeup. As you look at the following shots, compare this look to the variety of looks you can achieve with different lashes.

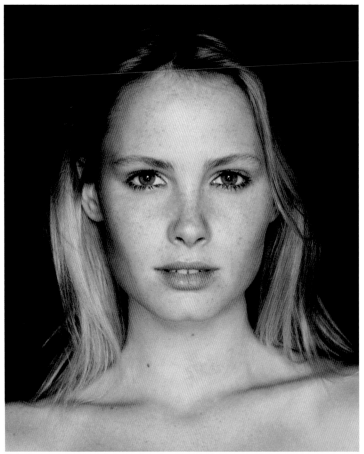

MODEL SHANAY HALL – VIVIEN'S MODEL MANAGEMENT **HAIR** MICHAEL WOLFF (MICHAEL WOLFF HAIR SALON)

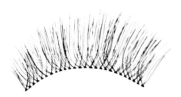

WISPY LASH

The first lash I've used is quite soft, and wispy on the ends. It has a clear lash line, giving a natural look. I like to use it on women who have never worn false eyelashes before. They're easy to apply and look fabulous.

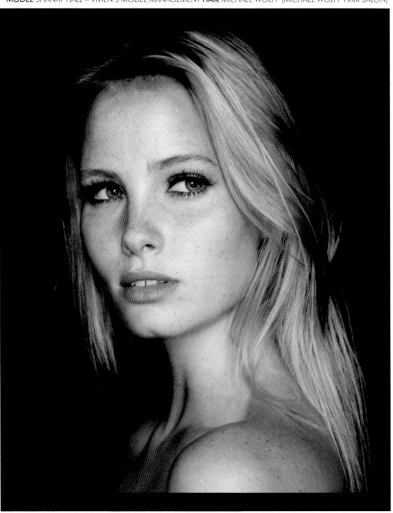

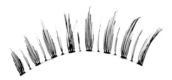

SEPARATED LASH

Similar to the 3/4 lash and easy to apply, the separated lash is great if you want your top lash to look more defined. Again, the base is clear, so it doesn't give you a heavy eyeliner effect.

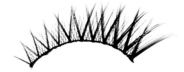

3/4 LASH

This 3/4 lash is the type I use most, as it fits every eyelid and is easy to apply. The base is black, so it will give you an eyeliner effect. However, because the lash only goes three-quarters of the way across your eyelid, you'll have to extend your eyeliner. I've smudged some black kohl pencil onto an angled brush and extended the line into the inner corner of each eye, as shown.

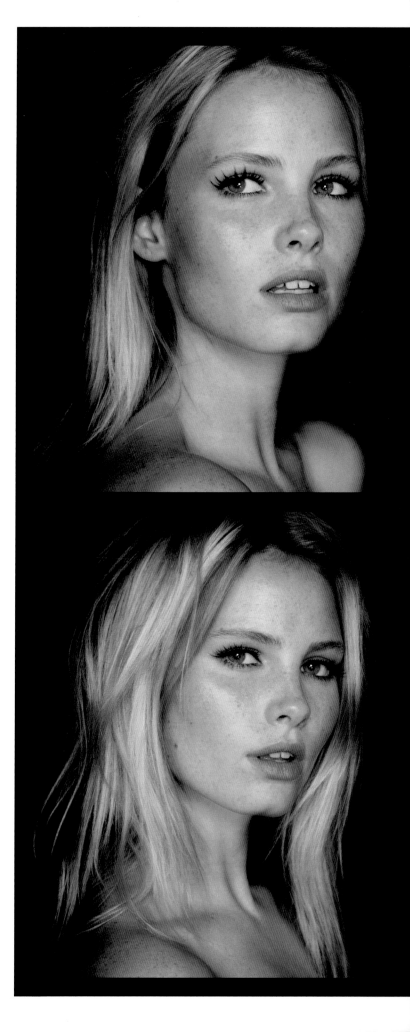

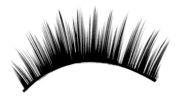

FULL LASH

This is one of the fullest lashes you can use—any fuller and you'll look like a drag queen. Before you apply it, check the length of the false lash against your natural eyelash line. If they differ in length, you may want to trim half a centimetre from the end of each lash before applying them. But if you want to go one step further, see below.

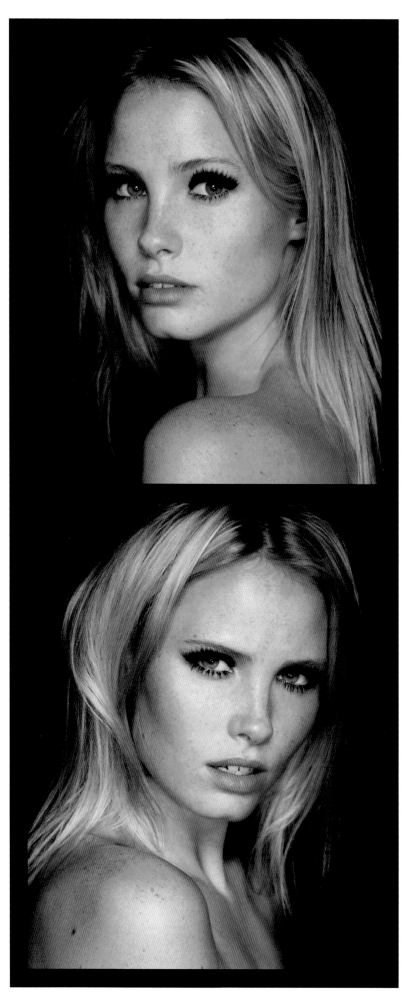

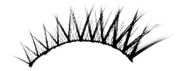

3/4 + MASCARA

This is exactly the same lash as the 3/4 one. All I've done is take the thickest black mascara I could find and apply five coats to the bottom lashes. Clump away!

5

EYE COLOUR CHARTS

YOUR EYES ARE NOT ONLY
THE WINDOWS TO YOUR
SOUL BUT ALSO THE FIRST
THING PEOPLE NOTICE.

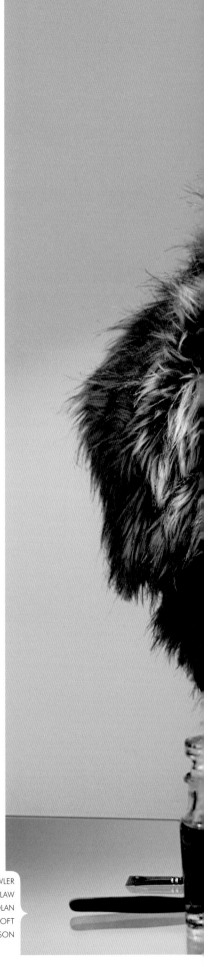

MODEL GEORGIA FOWLER
HAIR SARAH LAIDLAW
STYLING GEOFFREY NOLAN
ART DIRECTION BENJAMIN CROFT
MANICURE BELINDA JOHNSON

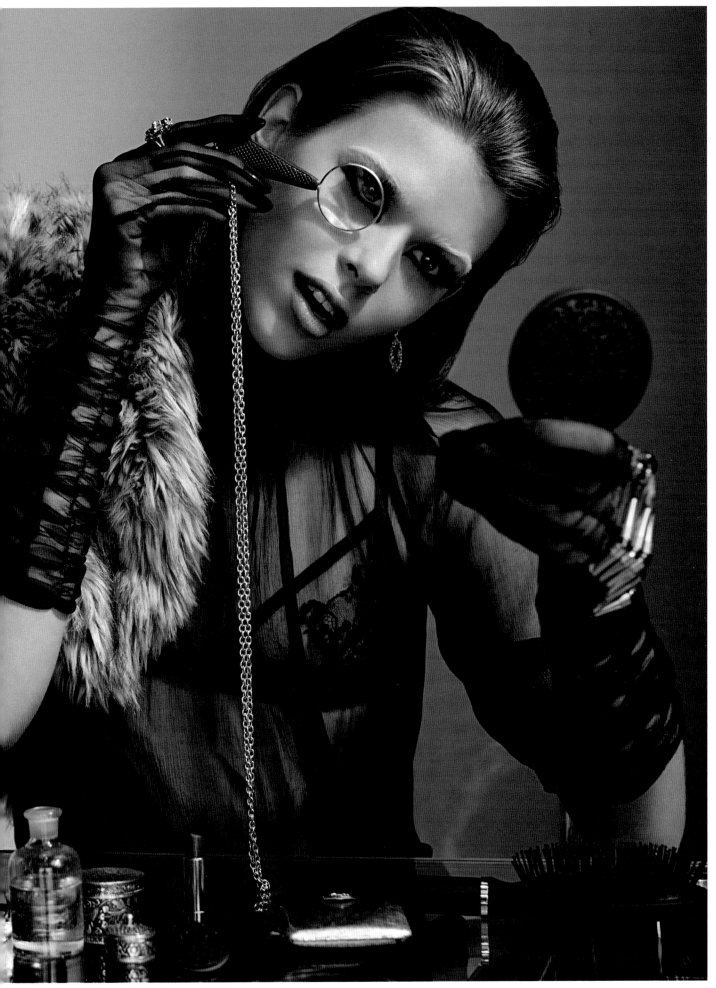

One of the best things you can do for your makeup is enhance your eyes. Even if you perfectly colour match your outfit, hat, shoes and accessories to your complexion, and your application is flawless, the wrong eye shadow can bring it all undone.

Sometimes even I get confused about the difference between someone being 'warm/cool' or 'summer/winter', as it's based on a combination of your skin, eyes and hair, and the three are not always the same tone. (You can have warm eyes with cool skin, or warm skin with cool hair.)

In *Makeup: The Ultimate Guide* (2008), I introduced you to colour expert Bronwyn Fraser, a successful personal stylist who has also worked for a leading global cosmetics company for many years. I regard her as my 'colour guru'. The two of us are constantly hired as consultants to help women get their colours right, and we've also conducted many seminars, workshops and events together.

On the following pages, we have revised and expanded the eye colour charts from *Makeup: The Ultimate Guide* to help you make colour choices quickly and easily. The natural eye colours have been grouped into both warm and cool. I've made these charts very easy to follow—simply locate your eye colour within one of the colour grids, and you'll find the perfect eye shadow colours for you.

Based on the fundamental rules of colour, the eye shadow charts are also divided into the following two groups:

1 colours that complement your natural eye colour; and

2 colours that intensify your natural eye colour and make it pop.

ALL EYE COLOURS

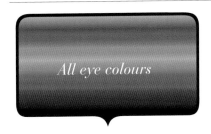

It's so simple. The chart on the right suits all eye colours, so I recommend you have two or three of these eye shadow colours in your makeup kit. If you have green eyes, just check the colour charts for green eyes on pages 54–5. On page 54 you'll find the perfect shades of green shadow to enhance or complement your eye colour. On page 55 are shades of violet that intensify your colour. As violet is opposite green on the colour wheel, your eyes will look greener than they've ever looked before. As we all know, opposites attract.

All the shades we've chosen can also be used as eyeliners, pencils or high-lighters, which come in either a matte or metallic finish. But please note: metallics enhance wrinkles, so stick to matte shades if you're concerned about fine lines.

From now on, make these charts your bible and never go shopping for makeup without them. This will also help you avoid feeling confused or overwhelmed by a sales consultant, who may be intent on recommending the 'colour of the season'.

Neutral

Eye shadow

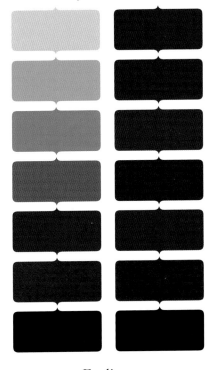

Eyeliners

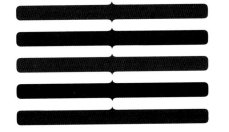

BLUE EYES

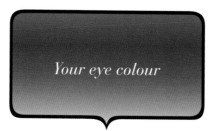

Your eye colour

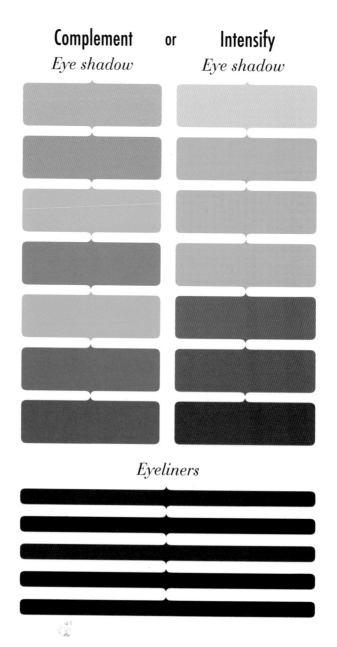

Complement or **Intensify**

Eye shadow   *Eye shadow*

Eyeliners

COOL BLUE

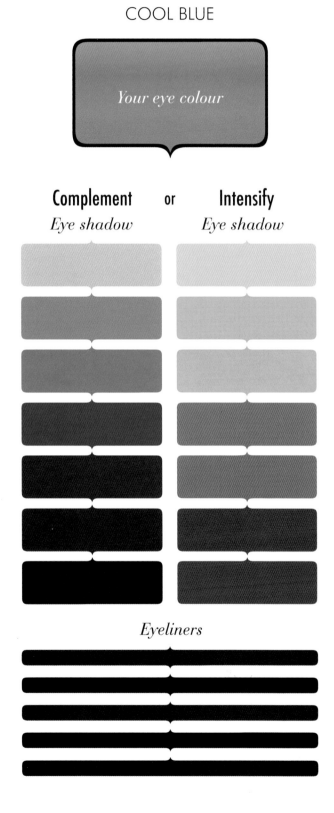

Your eye colour

Complement or **Intensify**

Eye shadow *Eye shadow*

Eyeliners

BROWN EYES

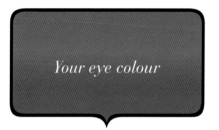

Your eye colour

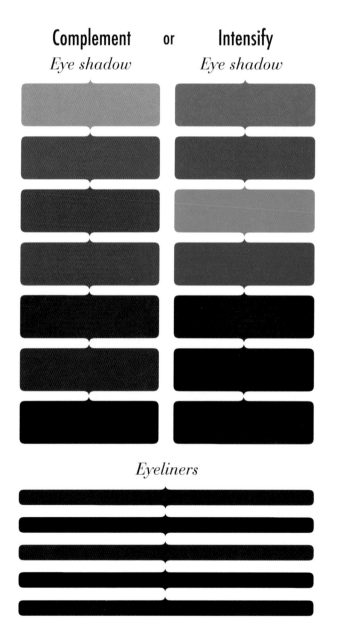

Complement	or	**Intensify**
Eye shadow		*Eye shadow*

Eyeliners

COOL BROWN

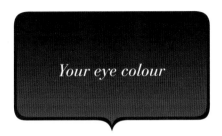

Your eye colour

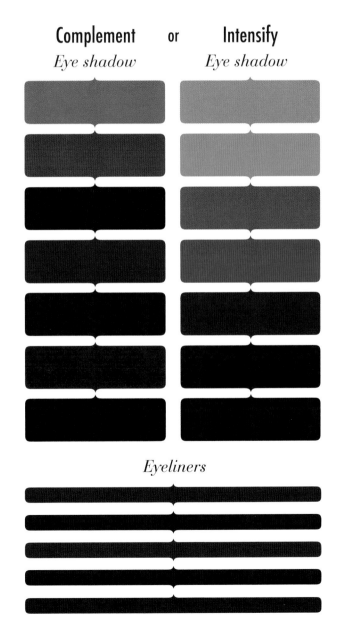

Complement	or	Intensify
Eye shadow		*Eye shadow*

Eyeliners

GREEN EYES

WARM GREEN

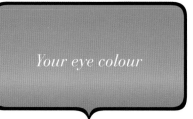

Your eye colour

Complement or **Intensify**

Eye shadow   *Eye shadow*

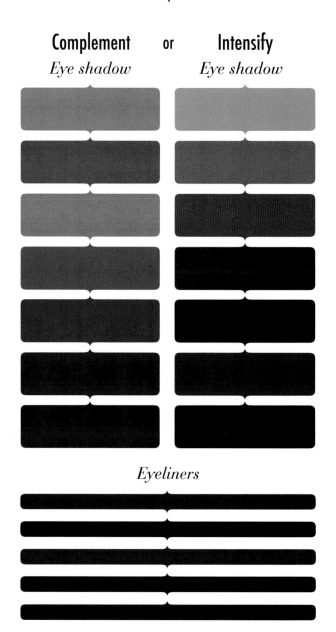

Eyeliners

COOL GREEN

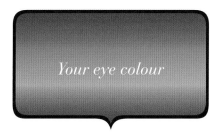

Your eye colour

Complement or **Intensify**

Eye shadow   *Eye shadow*

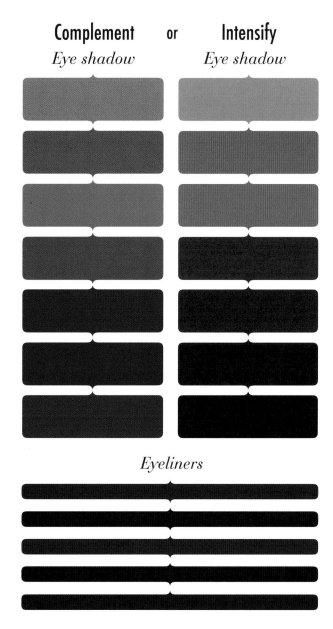

Eyeliners

HAZEL EYES

TRUE HAZEL

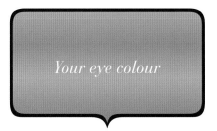

Your eye colour

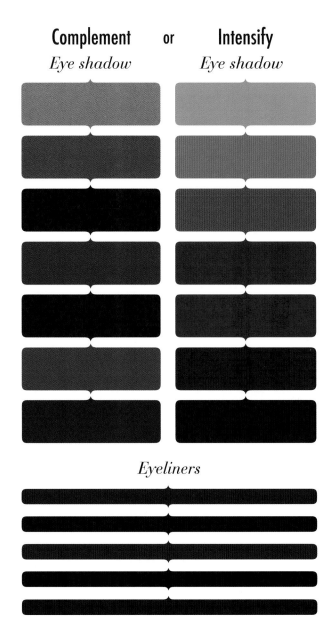

Complement or **Intensify**

Eye shadow   *Eye shadow*

Eyeliners

GOLDEN HAZEL

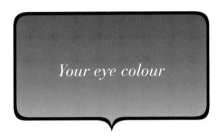

Your eye colour

Complement	or	Intensify
Eye shadow		*Eye shadow*

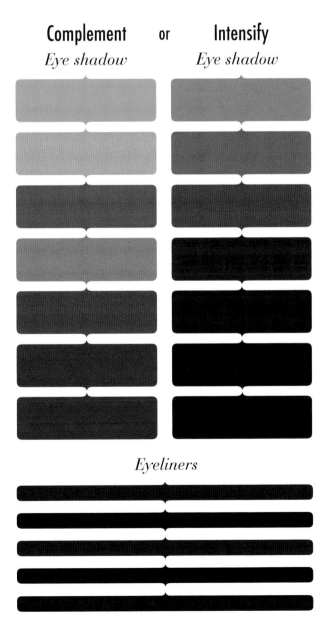

Eyeliners

6 EYEBROWS

YOUR EYEBROWS CAN BE YOUR
MOST POWERFUL ASSET AS WELL
AS MAKE OR BREAK YOUR MAKEUP.

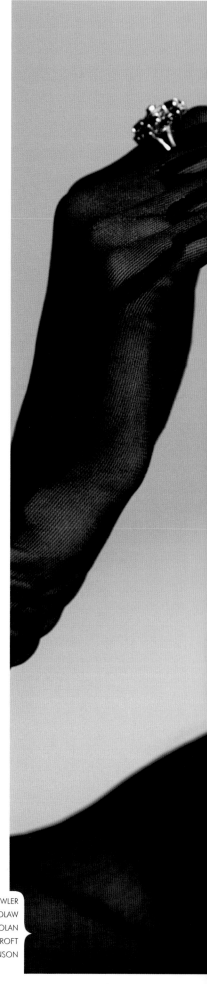

MODEL GEORGIA FOWLER
HAIR SARAH LAIDLAW
STYLING GEOFFREY NOLAN
ART DIRECTION BENJAMIN CROFT
MANICURE BELINDA JOHNSON

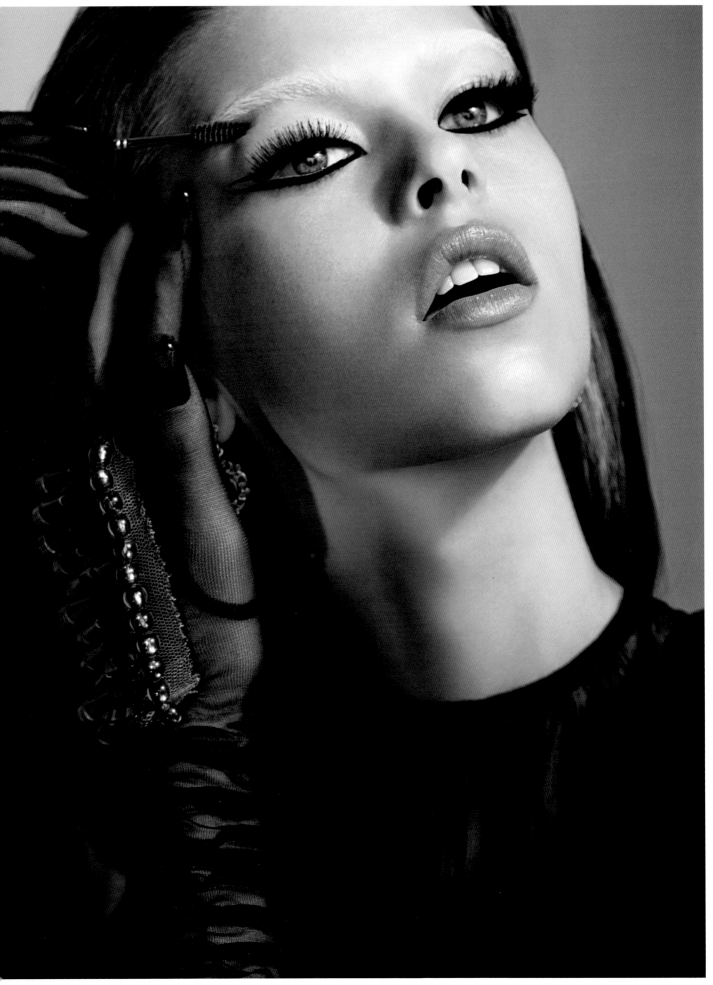

E

yebrows have the power to change your entire face, so treat them as an integral part of your face, not just an extra feature.

To demonstrate what I'm talking about, we took a photo of our model's eyebrows and changed them by computer to show you the three worst brow crimes you can commit (see the mug shots on page 62) before finishing with the perfect shape on page 64. This shape suits *every woman* on the planet, regardless of her age or race! And, yes, you too can have the perfect brow, be it thinner or fuller, but the critical factor is where your brow starts, lifts and ends!

As well as being an integral part of your face, your eyebrows change the shape of your nose like you wouldn't believe, as you can see in the photos on pages 62 and 64. Please take special note of these shots so you can identify the 'power of the brow'.

The higher you arch your brow, the older you look. Are you horrified, sitting there thinking, 'Oh no, that's me!'? It's so 1980s… need I say more? But as you can see in the first shot on page 62, over-arching your eyebrow creates a puffy eyelid that instantly ages you about ten years. Not only does it create lots of saggy space above your eyes, it also adds an instant 5 kilos (or more) to your face! So put your tweezers down and remember: when you straighten your brow and lower the arch, you create a younger, more sophisticated look.

If you have stray grey brow hairs, match the colour of your brows to your natural hair colour.

For an eyebrow overhaul, you'll need the following items:

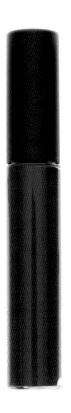

BROW MASCARA

This is a great little tool for temporarily lightening and darkening your brows. For the full rundown on brow mascara, see page 12.

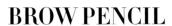

BROW PENCIL

If you use a brow pencil, make sure it exactly matches your brow colour. For a softer result, use eye shadows that match your brows.

TWEEZERS

A pair of scary pointed tweezers is my favourite, but they can be dangerous. Use the slanted ones we photographed in the 'Express makeup kit', page 12.

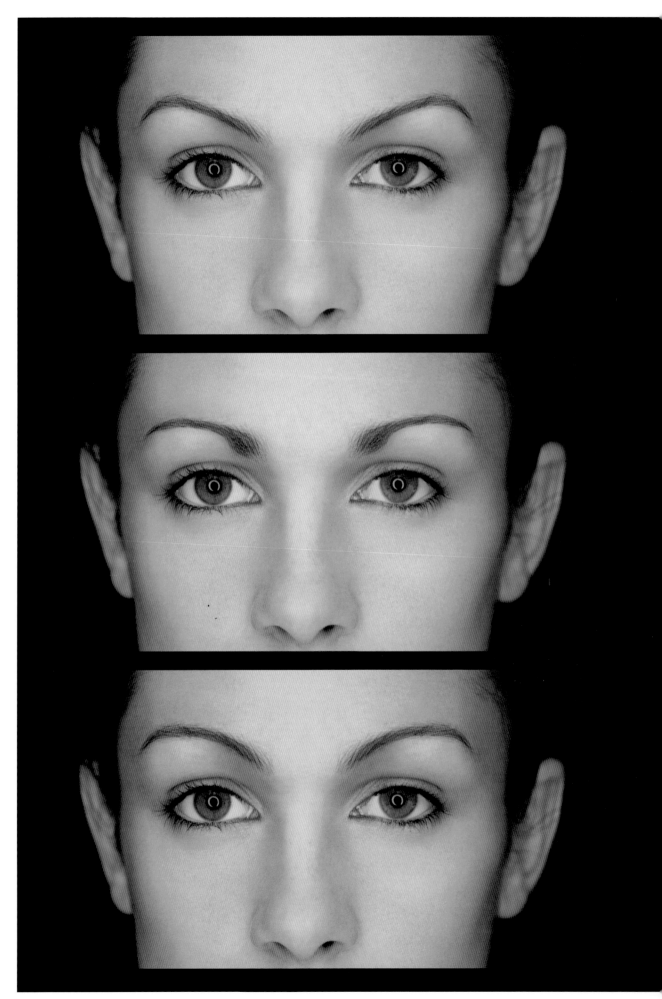

THE TRIANGLE

As you can see, a triangular-shaped brow gives you a natural frown that says 'I'm permanently annoyed' without even trying. Never angle your brows to this extreme. By lifting the brow at the dead centre of each eye, the downhill slant you create at the end of your brows is not only ageing but also creates a huge, saggy, puffy eyelid. Say to yourself, 'I shall not commit brow crime number one.'

THE TADPOLE

The tadpole brow creates a hard, angry, severe effect that looks 1980s and 1920s at the same time, and in an unflattering way—the further apart your brows are, the wider your nose looks.

This shape starts with a thick Brooke Shields brow, then suddenly changes into a thin pencil line. Whenever I see it, I shake my head and wonder why. And whenever I ask my makeup artist friends what brow shape is the hardest to work with, the tadpole wins hands down.

THE LETTER 'ᘻ'

It takes a lot of skill to get this shape so rounded, and never has so much effort gone into creating such an unflattering brow. This shape creates—yet again— unattractive puffy, droopy eyes.

If you want to immediately add years to your face, this is the number one brow shape. It just creates too much space between your lash line and your brows. It's also the worst shape if you have saggy, heavy lids. Only use it if you have a very flat eyelid, or if you're just addicted to the 'flapper' look from the 1920s and wear the polished, perfectly groomed makeup to match.

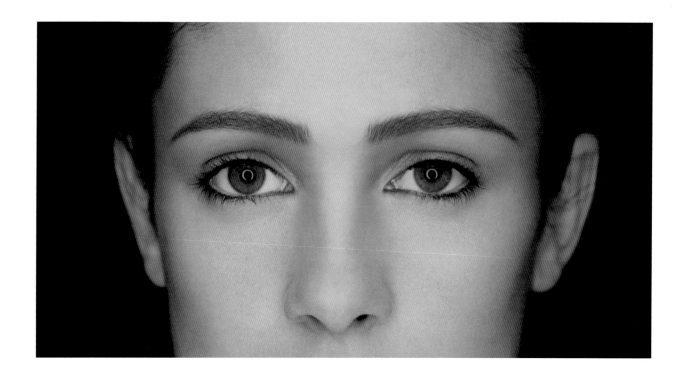

ACHIEVING THE PERFECT BROW

The perfect brow, with an arch that cuts through the brow bone, narrows and straightens your nose and lifts your eyes. As you can see in these two photos, the less you arch your brows, the younger you'll look.

Nose bridge line

Remember that myth your mother told you—start your brows by imagining a line from the outer edge of your nostrils to the inner corner of your eye? What if your nostrils are flared or wide? You'll be starting your brow halfway across your eye! Here's the rule: set the gap between your brows to match your desired nose bridge width, and you'll create the illusion of a thinner, more refined nose.

Brow starting point

Make sure the brow starting point is at a right angle. Keeping the bottom hairs on a perfect horizontal line here will not only lift your eyes but also stop everyone thinking you're in a bad mood. You may have to pluck any stray hairs under this line.

Brow arch point

The point where you should lift your brow is two-thirds of the way across your brow, in line with the outer edge of your iris. We've all been told never to pluck *above* our brows, but if you have stray hairs between your brow and your hairline, pluck away.

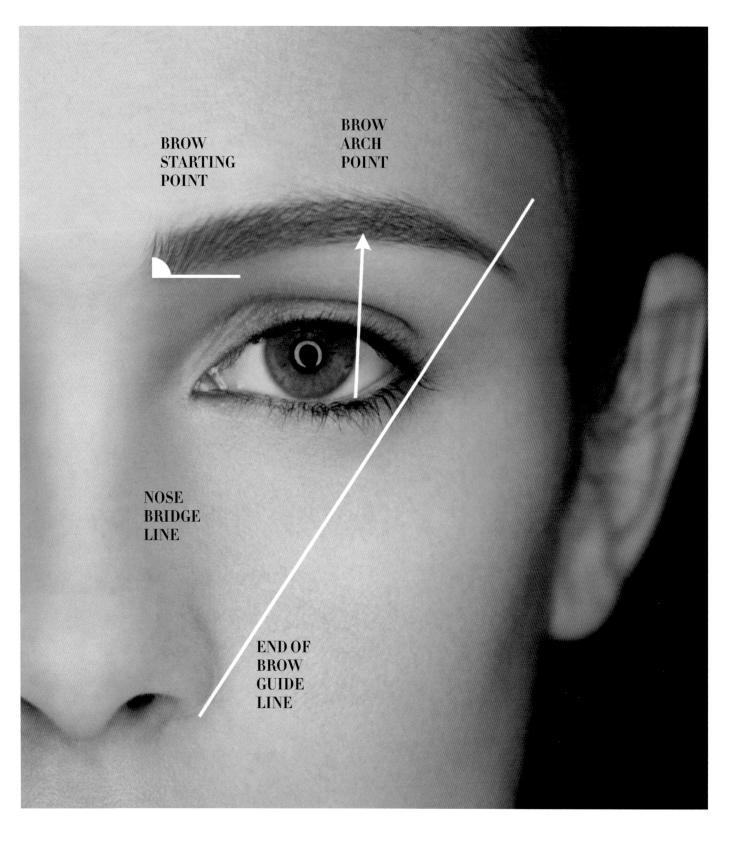

BROW
STARTING
POINT

BROW
ARCH
POINT

NOSE
BRIDGE
LINE

END OF
BROW
GUIDE
LINE

End of brow guide line

Imagine a line from the corner of your nose to the outer corner of your eye and out, then make sure your brows don't fall short of it, otherwise your eyes will look distorted and your brows will appear masculine and severe.

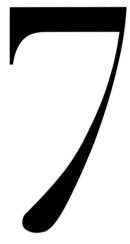

7 HIGHLIGHT

LUMINISE YOUR SKIN TO
GIVE IT A SUN-KISSED,
YOUTHFUL GLOW.

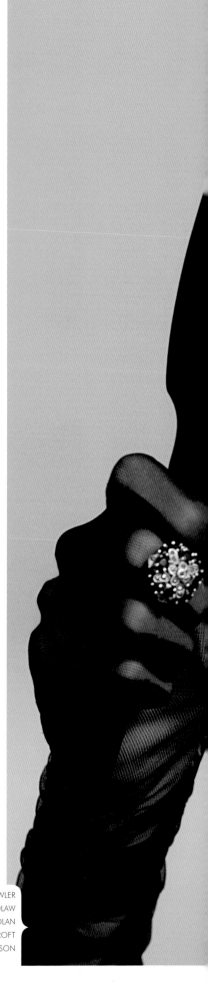

MODEL GEORGIA FOWLER
HAIR SARAH LAIDLAW
STYLING GEOFFREY NOLAN
ART DIRECTION BENJAMIN CROFT
MANICURE BELINDA JOHNSON

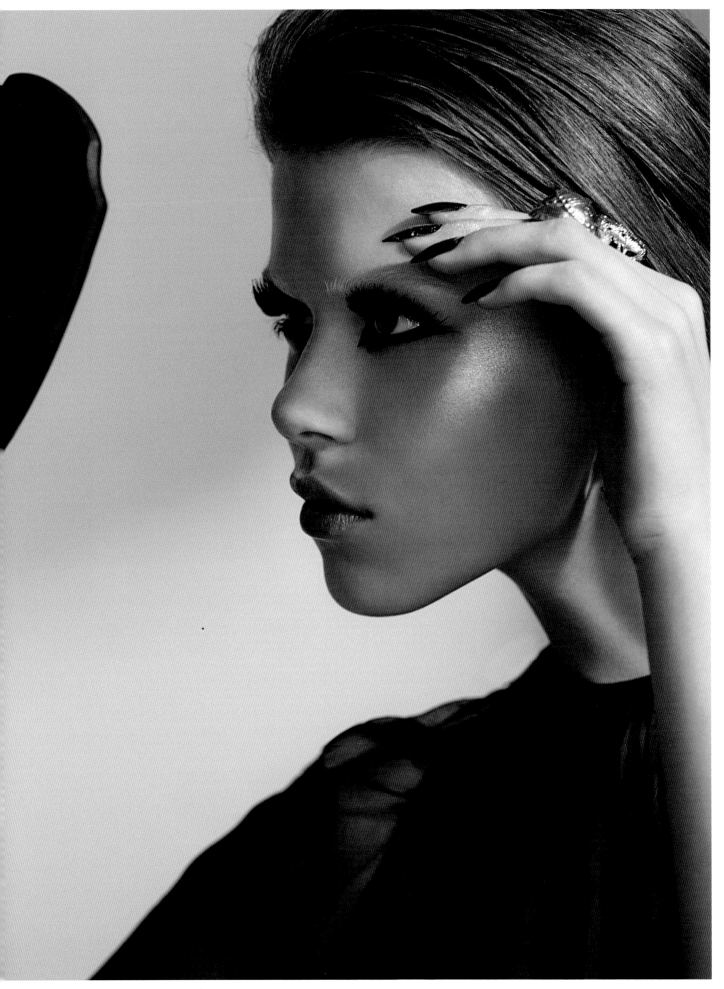

I highlight skin in one of the following two ways. One method is to mix a liquid highlighter (normally called luminiser) with foundation and apply it all over your face, which is fabulous for young and blemish-free skin. The other is to highlight only certain features. This gives your skin a hint of a glow while avoiding problem areas. There isn't a woman on this planet who doesn't want glowing, luminous, youthful skin. It's time to update your look.

Choosing highlighter colours

The best tip for choosing the right highlighter colour is to first apply the product to the cupid's bow on your top lip. You should see a natural shine, as if your natural skin tone is glowing, not colour. If it's too yellow, you've chosen a colour that's too dark for your skin tone. If it looks white and frosty, you've chosen a colour that's too light.

For example, for paler skin tones, use really sheer 'eggshell' soft gold pigments or creams.

For medium skin tones, use soft golds and rose golds, not bronzes.

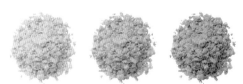

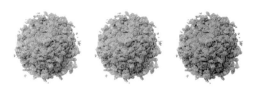

For dark skins, use deep golds and bronzes.

For black skins, use burgundies and dark, shimmery chocolate.

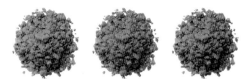

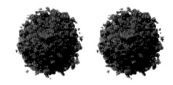

Highlighting dos and don'ts

Never use white or silver greys to highlight your skin. Only use these colours for highlighting the inner corners of your eyes.

When highlighting your cupid's bow, make sure this area is hair-free—girls, we don't highlight moustaches!

Avoid highlighters that reflect purple tones: always check your product on the back of your hand to make sure there are no purple/pink reflections, which are used in special effects to make actors look as if they're dead—obviously not a good look! These tones are hard to see but are very common in powdery mineral foundations.

If your brow is slightly hooded, or if you have a prominent brow bone, don't draw attention to this area by highlighting it. Here's the general rule: never highlight something you don't want people to look at!

Don't use cream highlighter on your eyelids—creams crease and eyelids move, so they're not a good combination. But creams are fabulous everywhere else.

Never use a frosty white eye shadow, and never ever highlight your whole brow bone, or it'll be 'Hello, soggy eyes!'

Where to highlight

These are the rules.

- *For youthful, wrinkle-free skin, you can luminise all over. Just add a few drops of luminising liquid to your base.*

- *If you're even slightly worried about fine lines and blemishes, follow the step-by-step technique on pages 72–4. You can choose to highlight all these areas shown in the photo opposite, or only a few.*

- *Just remember: don't use any of these highlighters on areas where your skin is extremely oily, blemished or lined.*

- *I believe everybody should highlight the inner corners of their eyes, which rarely wrinkle as we age. It's a great way to bring life and light into your eyes, and also to awaken tired eyes. However, it's essential to choose a highlighter that matches your skin tone.*

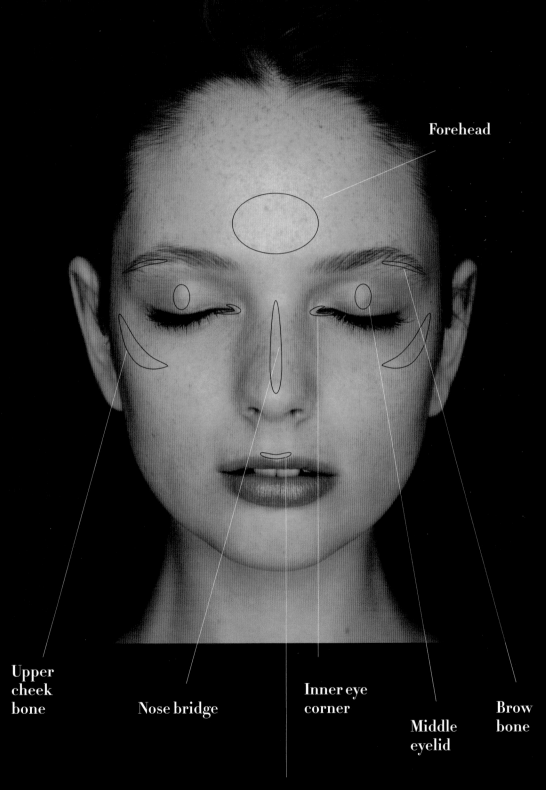

Forehead

Upper
cheek
bone

Nose bridge

Inner eye
corner

Middle
eyelid

Brow
bone

Cupid's bow

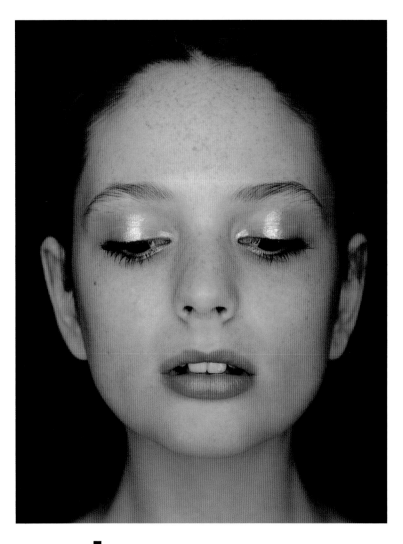

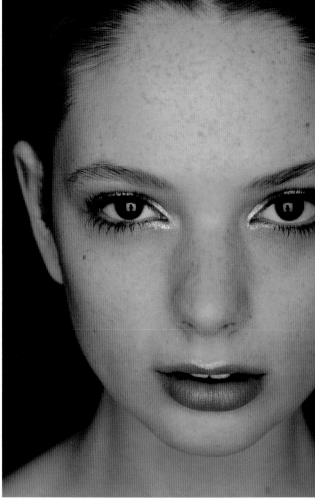

1 EYELIDS

To avoid fallout, wet an angle brush. Apply highlighter to the inner corners of your eyes, then look down and apply it to the centre of your eyelids.

2 CUPID'S BOW

Using the same wet brush, highlight your top lip, the cupid's bow. You can see how this instantly makes your lips fuller without you having to obviously overdraw your lip line.

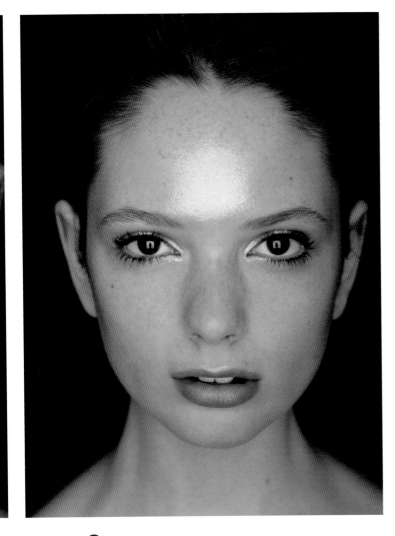

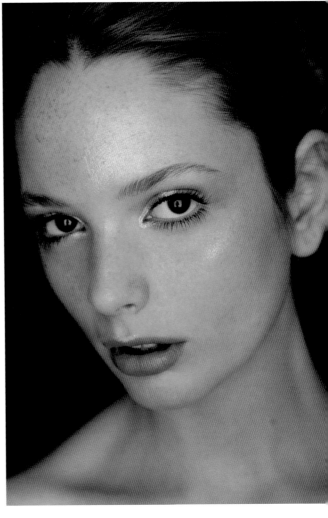

3 NOSE

Highlight down the centre of your nose, but be careful not to go to the very tip. (If you're over-oily in this area, don't highlight your nose at all.)

4 FOREHEAD

With a kabuki brush, apply highlighter to the centre of your forehead. This gives the very youthful illusion of a rounded forehead, and is great for normal to dry skin; again, avoid this area if it is oily.

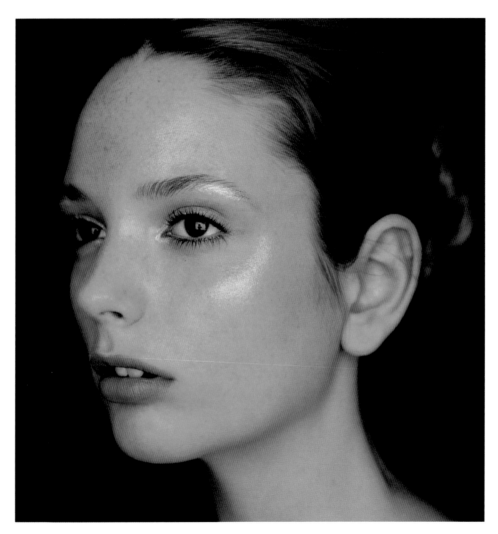

5 CHEEKS & BROWS

Using your fingertip or a fan brush, apply a hint of highlighter to your cheekbone. You should only be able to see this highlight when you turn side on. If you can see it front on, you've used too much. Avoid this area if you're heavily lined. Wetting a fine angle brush, highlight very closely along the last third of your eyebrow. Keep this section very thin so you don't create a puffy eyelid. Highlighting the whole brow bone creates an ageing effect.

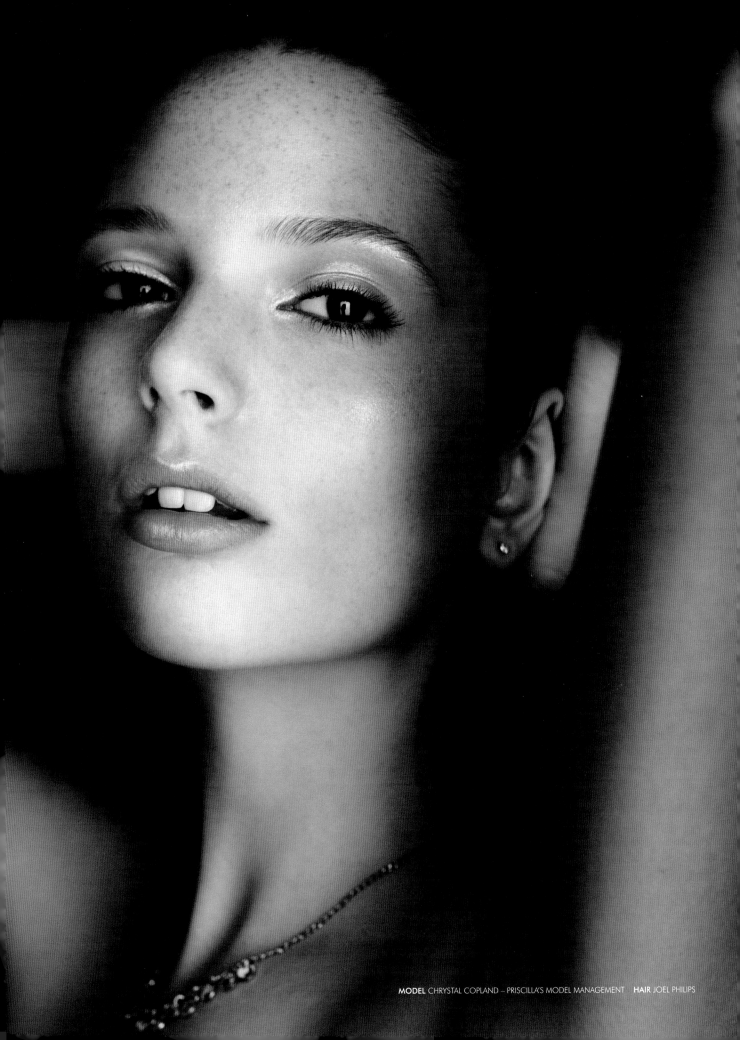

8

EXPRESS LOOKS

HERE ARE LOTS OF KILLER
LOOKS THAT YOU CAN
PULL OFF FAST.

MODEL GEORGIA FOWLER
HAIR SARAH LAIDLAW
STYLING GEOFFREY NOLAN
ART DIRECTION BENJAMIN CROFT
MANICURE BELINDA JOHNSON

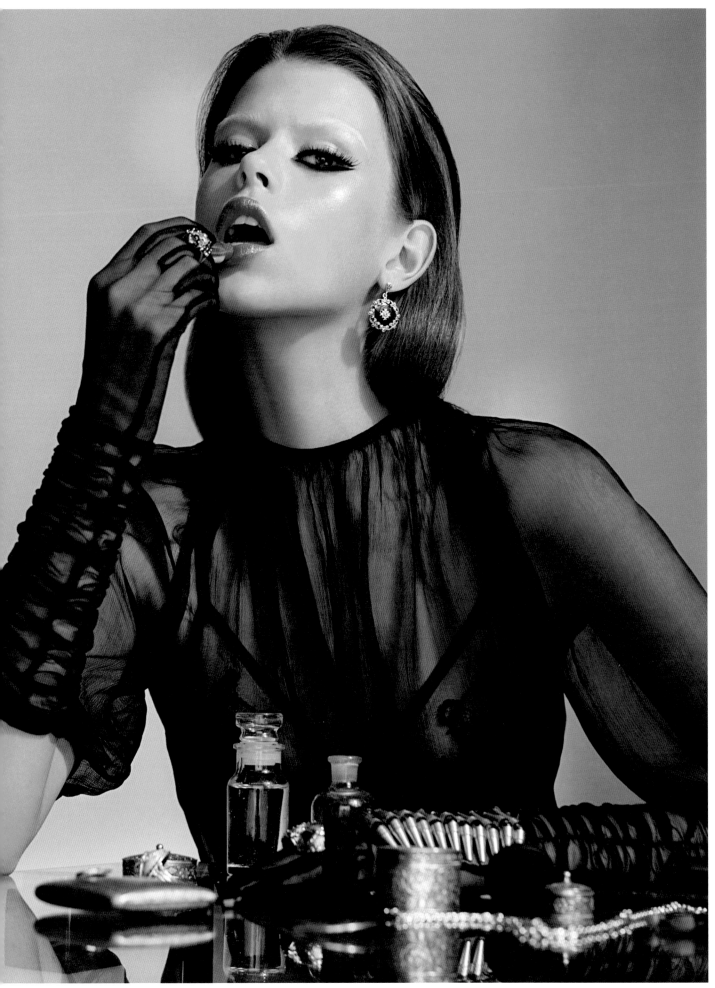

1 | NATURAL GLAMOUR

A CLEAR VERSATILE LOOK
THAT SUITS ALL SKIN TONES.

1 PREP & FOUNDATION

Prep your skin, then
apply light foundation
and concealer. For a
velvety finish, add light
translucent powder.
Finish by applying a
mineral powdered blush
with a kabuki brush.

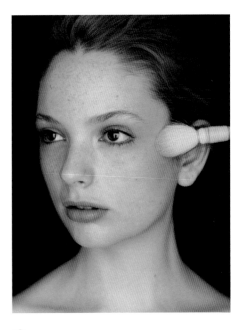

2 LASHES

Curl your eyelashes,
then apply lots of black
mascara to your top and
bottom lashes.

3 LIPS

Apply a red lipstick that
suits your skin tone—
for example, orange-reds
can make your teeth look
yellow, while burgundy-
reds make your teeth
look whiter.

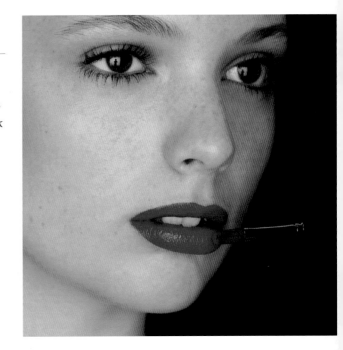

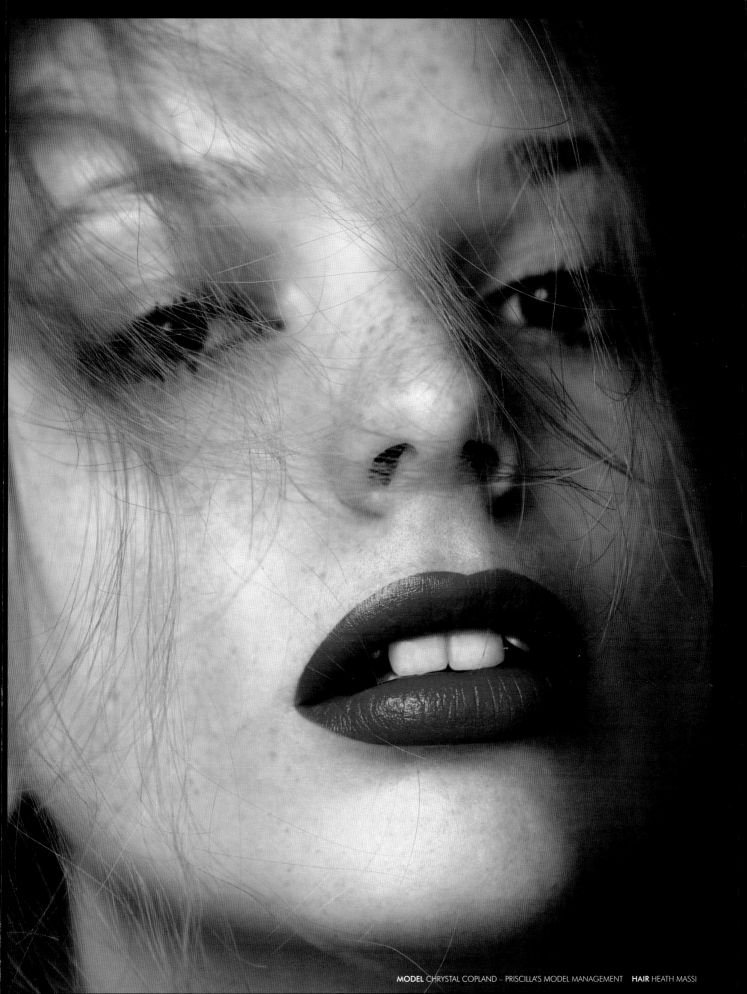

2 | AUBERGINE VELVET

RICH VIOLET WITH THE
DEFINITION YOU GET
FROM A SMOKY EYE.

1 EYE PREP & FOUNDATION

Prep your skin, making
sure you remove all the
oil from your eyelids.
Apply foundation to your
eyelids only, then lightly
powder them.

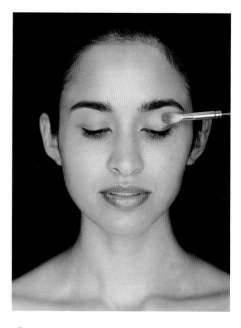

2 EYE SHADOW

Now apply a rich violet pigment to each
eyelid, blending to just under the brow
bone. Ignore the messy fallout, which
you can clean up later. To intensify the
colour, wet your brush.

3 UPPER DEFINITION & BLENDING

Use black eye shadow or gel
eyeliner to blend the socket
line. For better blending,
apply gentle pressure and
extend the line outwards
as shown.

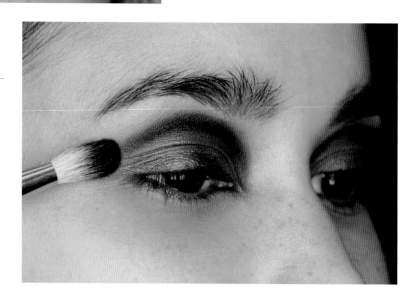

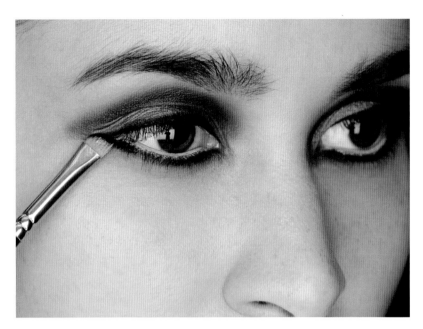

4 LOWER DEFINITION & BLENDING

With a fine angle brush, apply black gel eyeliner along the lower and upper lash lines, and softly blend. Then use a creamy white pencil to line inside your inner eyelids.

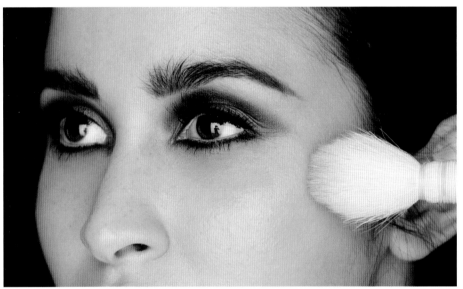

5 FINISHING EYES & FOUNDATION

Use a baby wipe to clean up any eye shadow fallout from under your eyes, then apply foundation mixed with a luminiser. Define your eyebrows. Curl your lashes and apply lots of black mascara. Apply a cream coral blush.

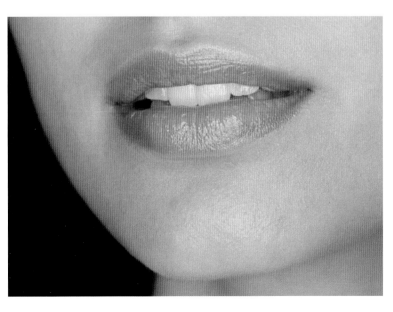

6 LIPS

Finish with a matching coral lipstick.

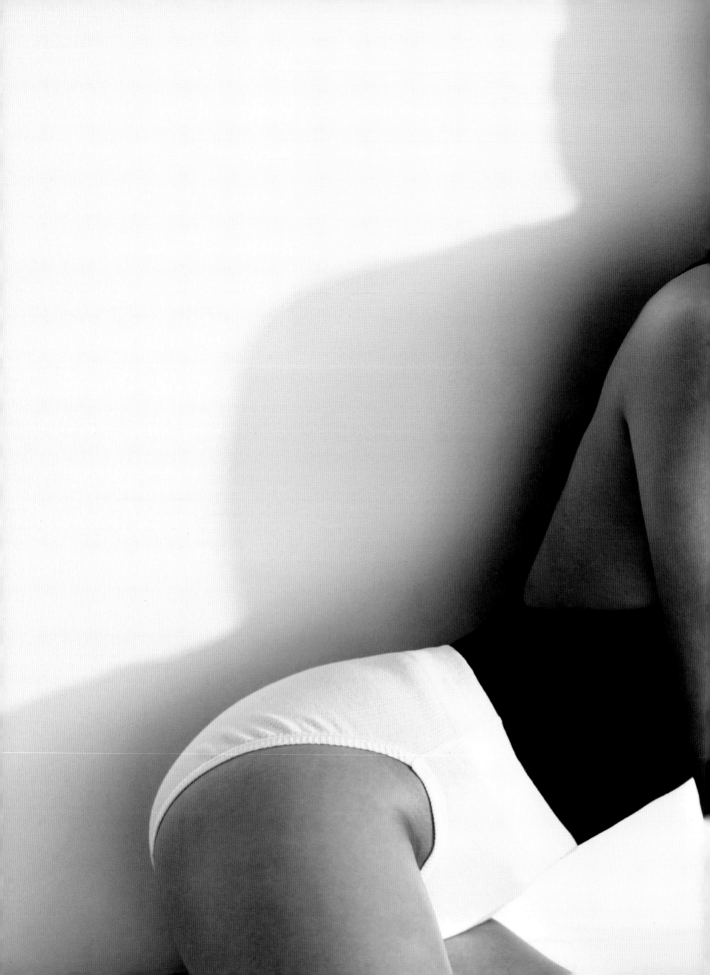

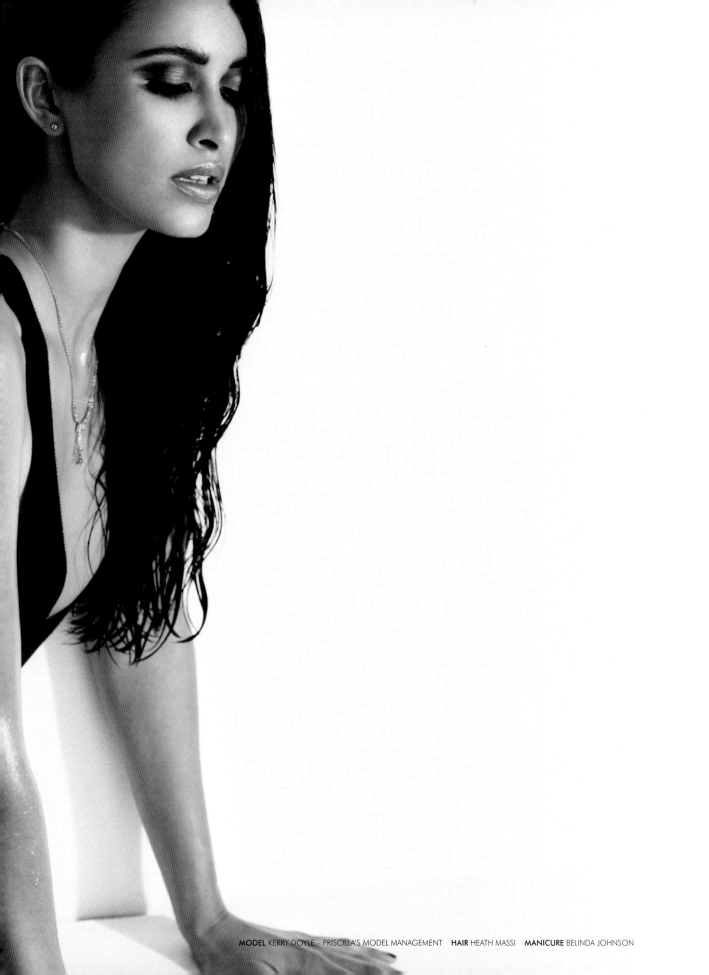

3 | SOFT CORAL

SOFT SHADES THAT SUIT
ALL SKINS AND ALL AGES.
A DIVINE DAY LOOK.

1 PREP & FOUNDATION

Prep your skin, then
apply liquid foundation
all over your face,
powdering your eyelids
only. Then take a soft,
pink blush and apply it
to your eyelids and along
the bottom lash line.

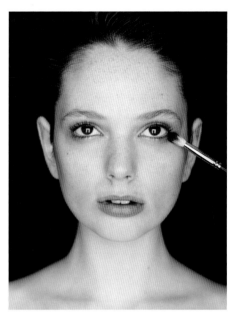

2 CHEEKS & LIPS

Use a kabuki brush
to apply a cream coral
blush to your cheeks
and lips. This will give
them a luminous texture.

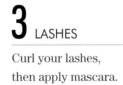

3 LASHES

Curl your lashes,
then apply mascara.

*If your eyes are looking tired, apply creamy
white pencil to the inner rims of each eye.*

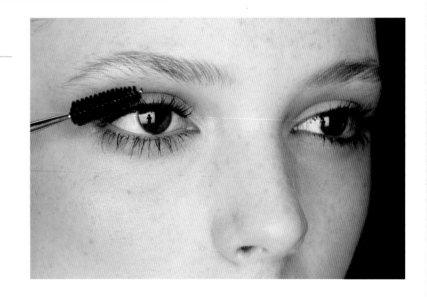

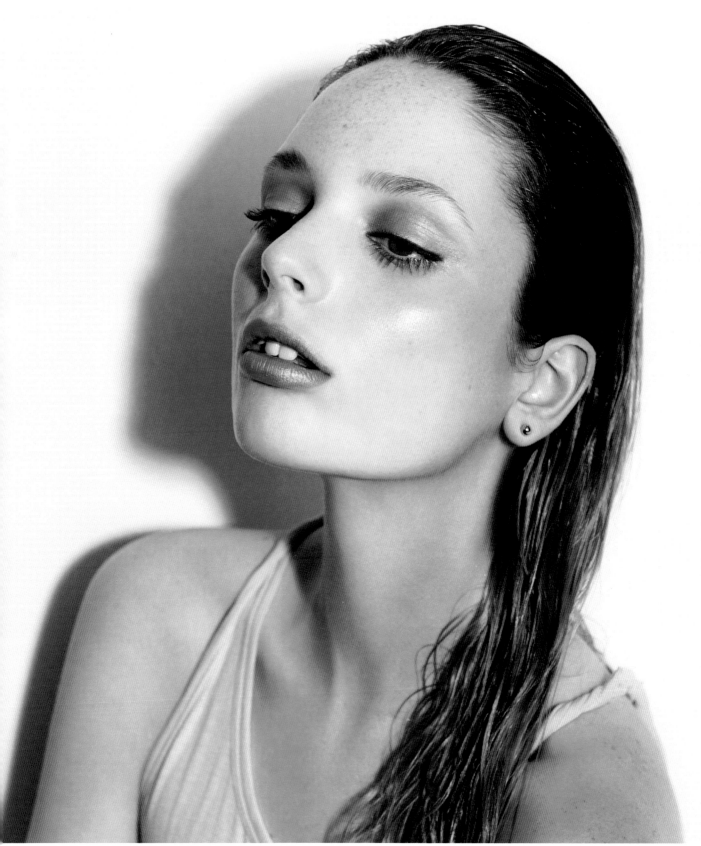

MODEL CHRYSTAL COPLAND – PRISCILLA'S MODEL MANAGEMENT   **HAIR** HEATH MASSI

4 | LUSH BLUSH

A FEMININE, SULTRY EYE THAT ALL WOMEN DESIRE.

1 PREP & FOUNDATION

Apply foundation all over your face, then lightly powder all over, including your eyelids. Groom and define your eyebrows (see 'Achieving the perfect brow', page 64).

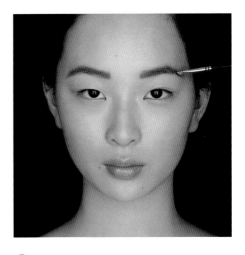

2 LOWER DEFINITION

Apply a chocolate-brown pencil to your outer bottom lash lines, then blend with a chocolate-brown eye shadow.

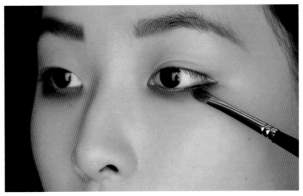

3 EYE SHADOW

Smudge pencil on your outer top lash lines. Look straight ahead and apply the same chocolate-brown eye shadow to your upper lids. Fill in the lids later. Blend at the edges with translucent powder.

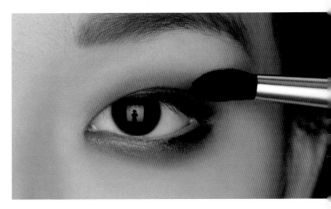

4 LASHES, CHEEKS & LIPS

Curl your eyelashes, then apply mascara and false separated lashes. Use a kabuki brush to apply blush to your cheeks. Finish off with a soft apricot blush and lip balm on your lips.

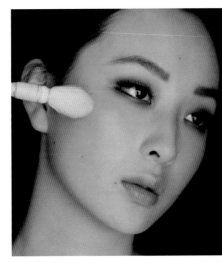

Add a soft highlight to your nose and to the cupid's bow on your top lip (see 'Highlight', pages 72–3).

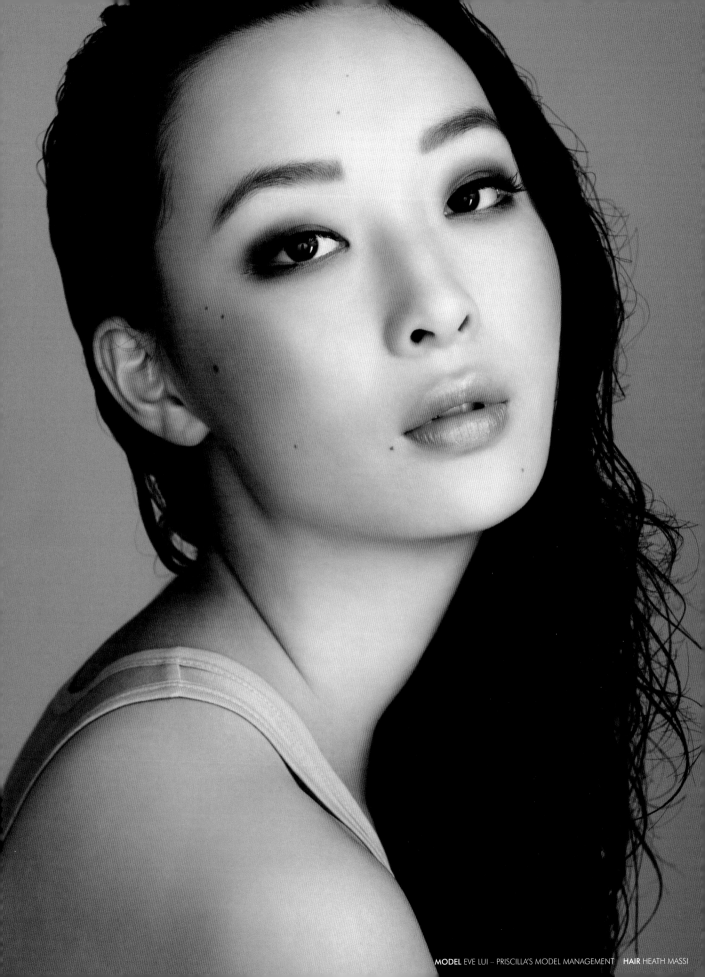

5 | COCO DESIRE

THE QUICK WAY TO APPLY
THE CLASSIC CAT EYE.

1 FOUNDATION & BLUSH

Define your brows, and
apply sheer foundation
before lightly powdering
your entire face. Apply a
soft beige blush to your
cheeks, and a wash of
blush over your eyelids.

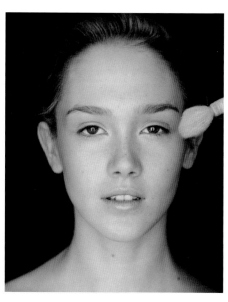

2 EYE SHADOW

Using an eye shadow
brush, do a soft wash
of a matte taupe—
think matte brown—
eye shadow around
your entire eye. Repeat
for the other eye. Do
most of this looking
straight ahead, as you
want this colour to
lightly creep up under
your brow bone.

*Keep a clean brush with translucent powder on standby to help you blend.
When smudging kohl pencil on your eyelids, turn the brush upside down.
This keeps the intensity along the lash lines, giving you a stronger effect.*

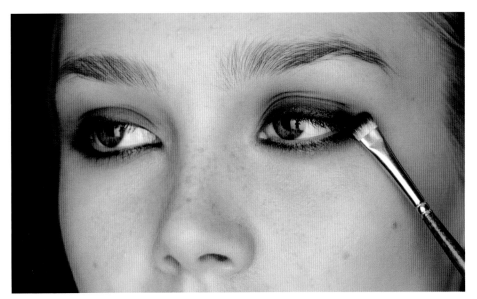

3 UPPER & LOWER DEFINITION

Using a chocolate-brown pencil, smudge around the entire lash line, top and bottom, then blend with the mini square blending brush. Repeat for the other eye.

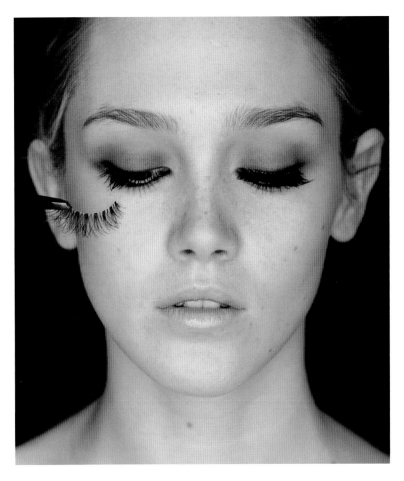

4 LASHES, BROWS & LIPS

Curl your lashes, and apply lots of black mascara to the top lashes only, then apply false wispy lashes. This will give you more of a cat-eye effect. Finish the look with a nude lipstick and, finally, add a defined, filled-in brow.

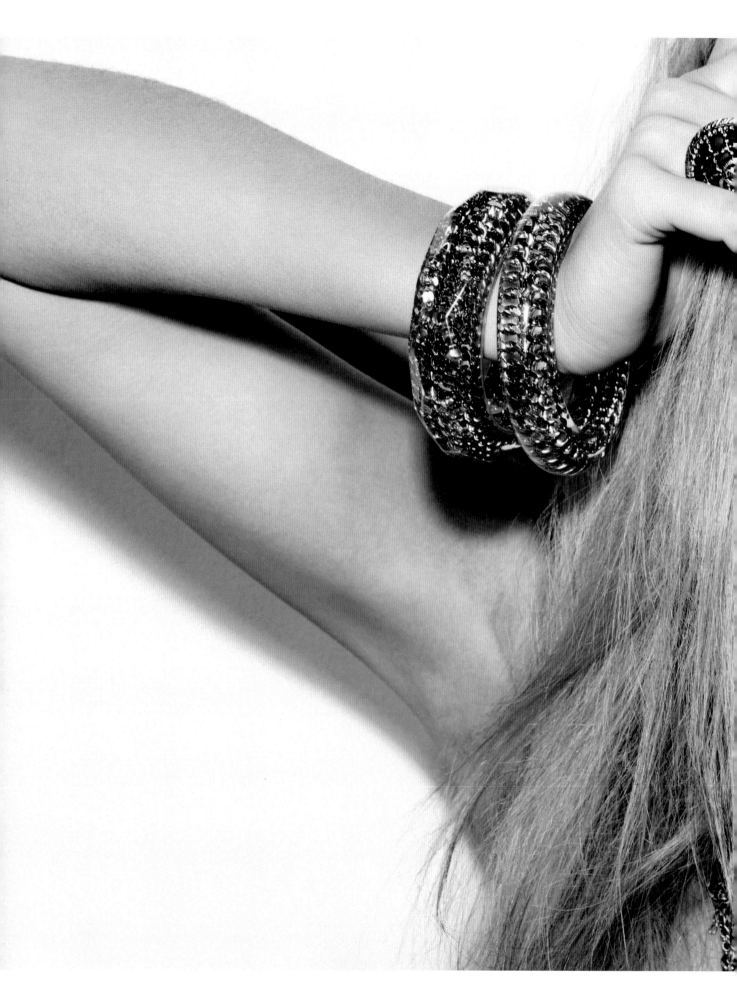

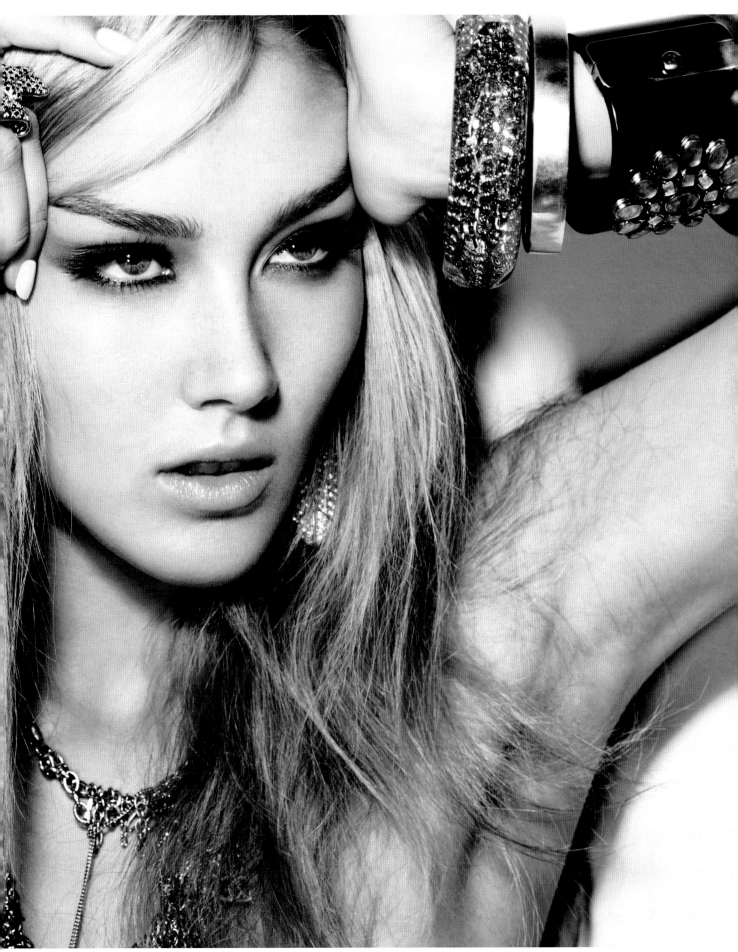

6 | PLATINUM NOIR

A SIMPLE EYE TO
COMPLEMENT A
POWERFUL POUT.

1 FOUNDATION & EYE PREP

First, apply cream
foundation, then lightly
powder your eyelids only
and highlight your skin.
Use a cream-coloured
pencil to line the inner
rims of your eyes.

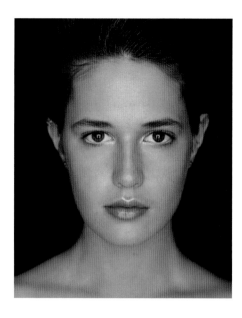

2 EYE SHADOW

Apply a matte cream-
beige eye shadow.

3 BLENDING

Looking straight ahead,
apply a matte aubergine
eye shadow to the inner
corner of each eye, then
blend it straight across
your brow bone.

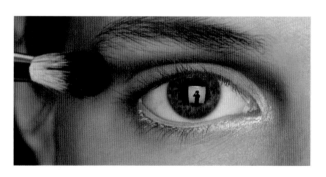

4 LASHES, LIPS & CHEEKS

Curl your lashes, then
apply lots of mascara to
the top lashes only. Apply
a dark lipstick, and finish
by shading under your
cheekbones. The model
accidentally wiped her
top lip during the shoot,
so she has a faded upper
lip line in the finished shot.
I love it...

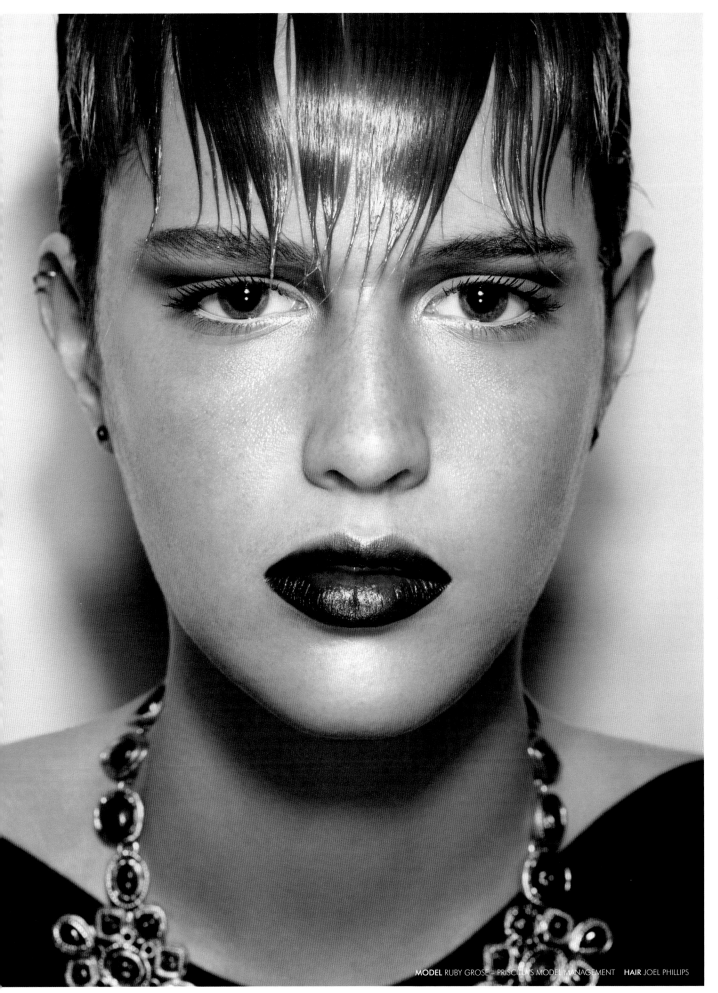

7 LINED & LACQUERED

A FOOLPROOF WAY
TO CREATE THE PERFECT
RAZOR-SHARP EYE.

1 FOUNDATION & EYELINER

Groom and lightly fill your brows. Apply foundation and concealer, then lightly powder your face. Apply slightly tacky sticky tape under each eye (stick it to an item of clothing a few times so it loses some of its adhesive), then apply a black gel eyeliner.

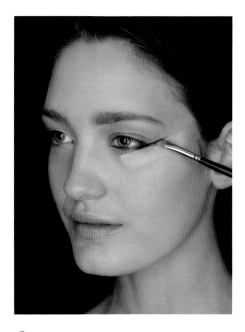

2 EYELINER

Apply lots of kohl pencil to the inner rim of each eye. Tape your eyelids as shown (see also Look 24, page 134) and colour in with a black eye gel. Take it along your entire top eyelash line, then peel off the tape.

3 LASHES, LIPS & CHEEKS

Curl your lashes, then go to town with mascara on both your top and bottom lashes—the clumpier the better. Apply a soft, nude lip gloss and a hint of blush.

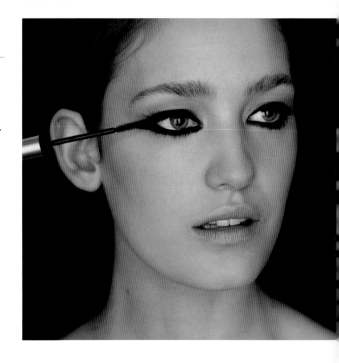

If you're clumping your lashes, go all out, or they'll just look like unfinished dirty lashes.

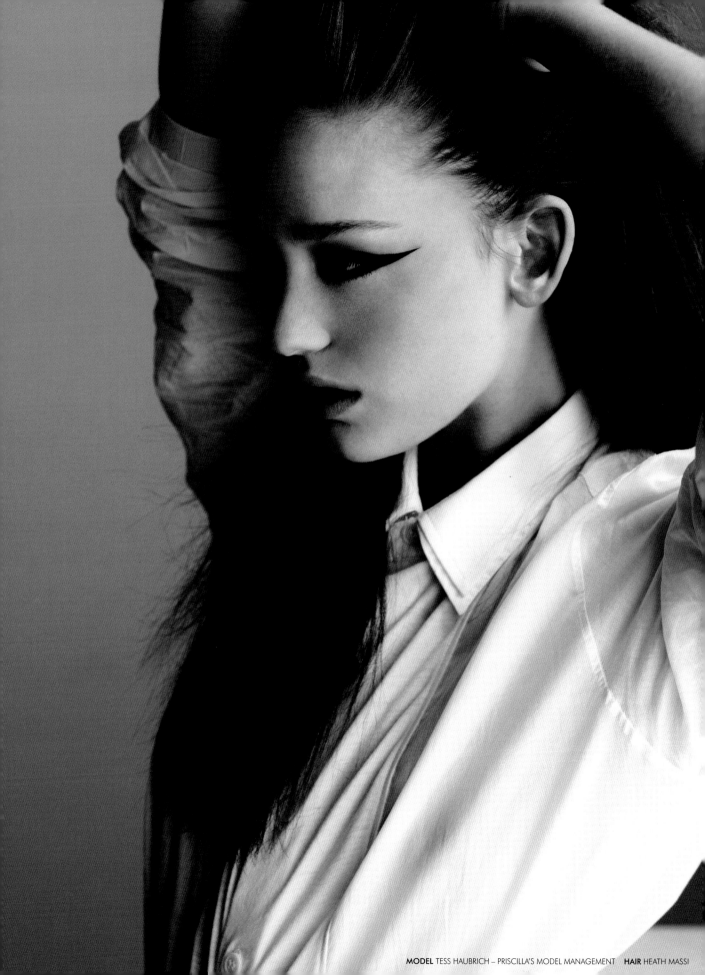

8 | PASTEL BOMB

CREAMY SKIN, PEACHY
SHADES, DAY OR NIGHT.

1 BRONZER & HIGHLIGHTER

This look requires bronzer (see page 38), so I'm using a foundation four shades darker than the model's natural skin tone. Only do this if your body is tanned or dark/olive (the model had a spray tan). After bronzing, highlight your skin and groom your brows.

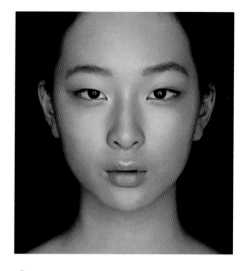

2 EYE SHADOW

While looking straight ahead, use a bright metallic orange eye shadow around the whole of each eye, then blend the outer edge with a soft coral pink.

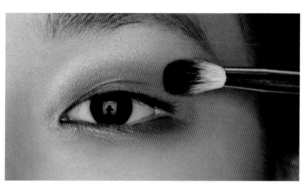

3 EYES & CHEEKS

Apply a creamy white pencil to the inner rim of each eye. After curling your lashes, add black mascara and false 3/4 lashes. Finally, apply metallic peach blush to each cheek. Eye shadow pigments are also great for this.

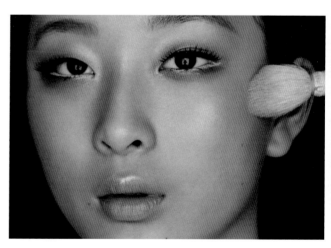

4 LIPS

Apply a soft, sheer baby-pink lip gloss.

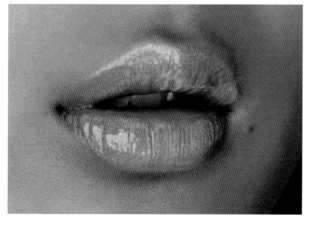

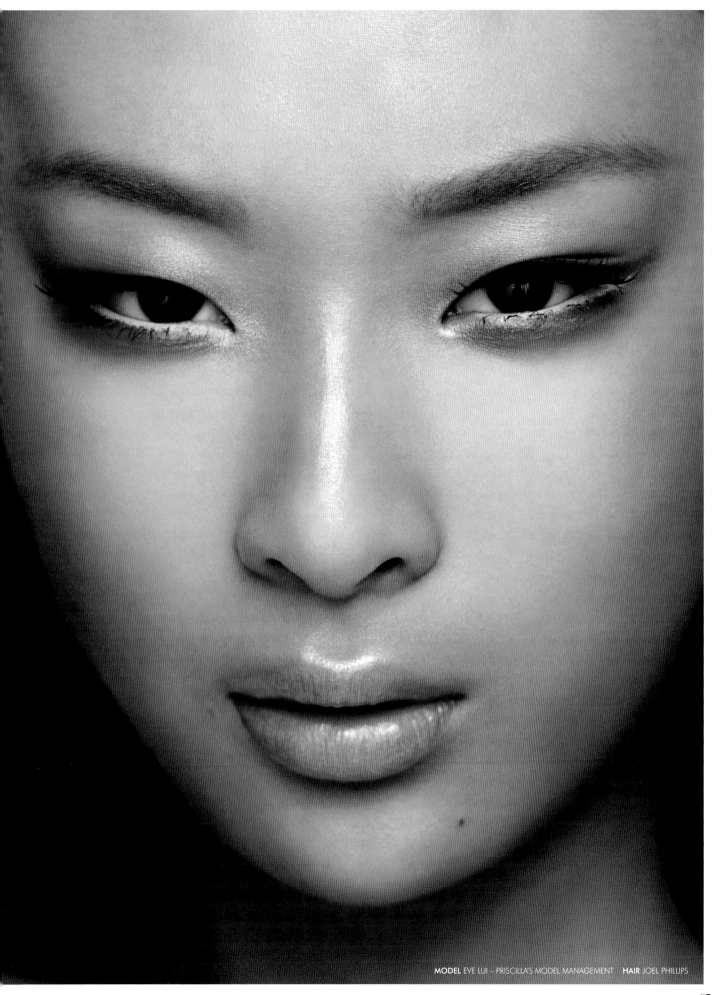

MODEL EVE LUI – PRISCILLA'S MODEL MANAGEMENT   **HAIR** JOEL PHILLIPS

9 BARE NATURALE

THE NATURAL LOOK
WITH A FABULOUS TWIST.

1 BROWS

Using a *gentle* facial bleach, I've lightened the model's eyebrows, something you should allow only a *professional* to do. If you do it yourself, you risk ending up with bright orange brows.

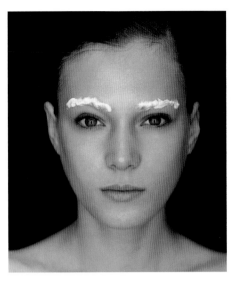

2 FOUNDATION & LASHES

Apply foundation all over your face, except your eyelids. This produces a glossy eye effect, one of my favourite looks. Unfortunately, it doesn't last long, so you'll need to maintain it (keep a mirror handy). Curl your lashes, and apply loads of mascara to both the top and bottom lashes.

3 EYELIDS & CHEEKS

To set off this look, matte down your foundation, using either powder or an anti-shine primer (see page 32), and apply a soft baby-pink lip gloss to your eyelids. Again, you'll need to smooth this out after a while, as nothing can make lip gloss last. Apply a cream blush to your cheeks.

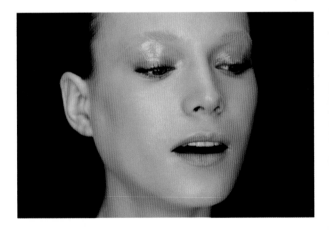

4 LIPS

Finish off with a soft peach-cream lipstick.

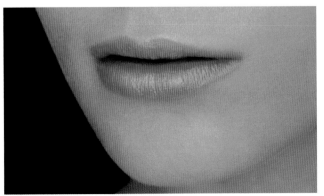

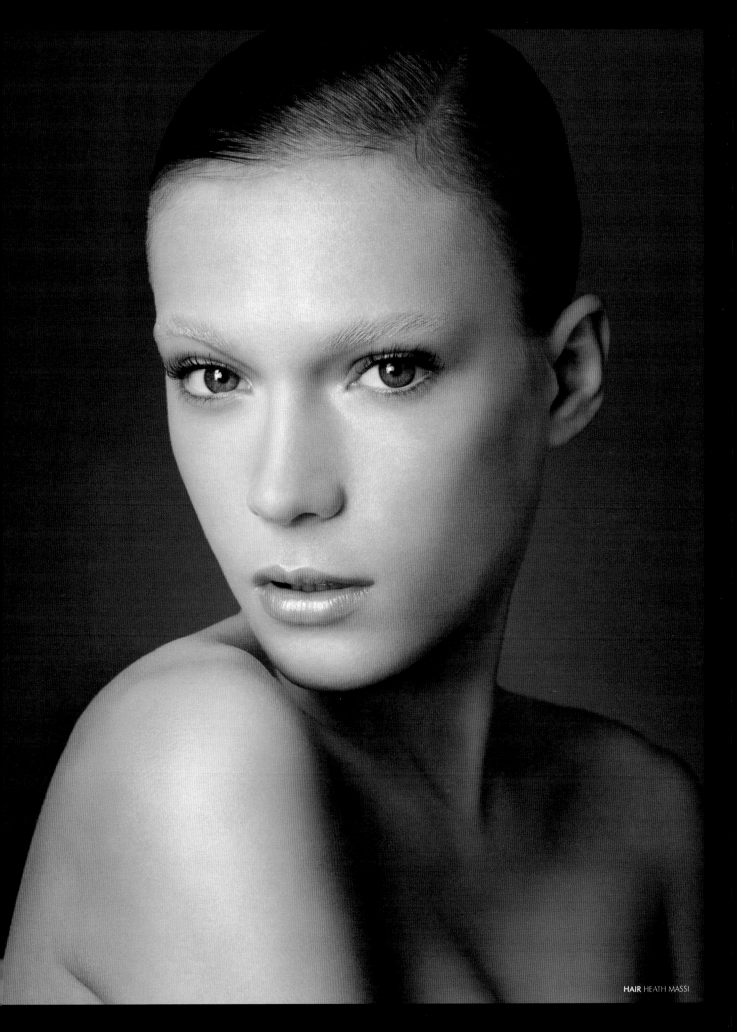

10 | PRETTY IN PINK

A SOFT, FEMININE AND FLATTERING STYLE.

1 PREP, DEFINITION & FOUNDATION

Prep your face and eyelids. Lightly powder your eyelids, then apply a soft matte taupe-brown eye shadow to your eyelids as well as softly under each eye. Trace around the entire lash line with a brown pencil, and blend. Clean up any fallout, and apply a liquid foundation before lightly powdering your face.

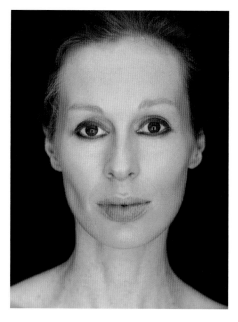

2 LASHES & BROWS

Curl your lashes, then apply lots of black mascara and false 3/4 lashes to your top lashes only. Define and extend your eyebrows.

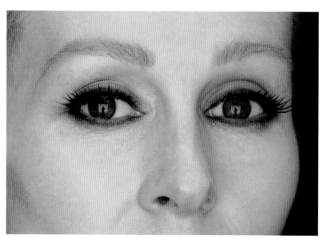

3 CHEEKS & LIPS

Apply a soft orange blush and a nude- or bone-coloured lipstick.

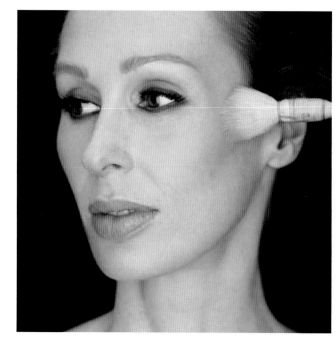

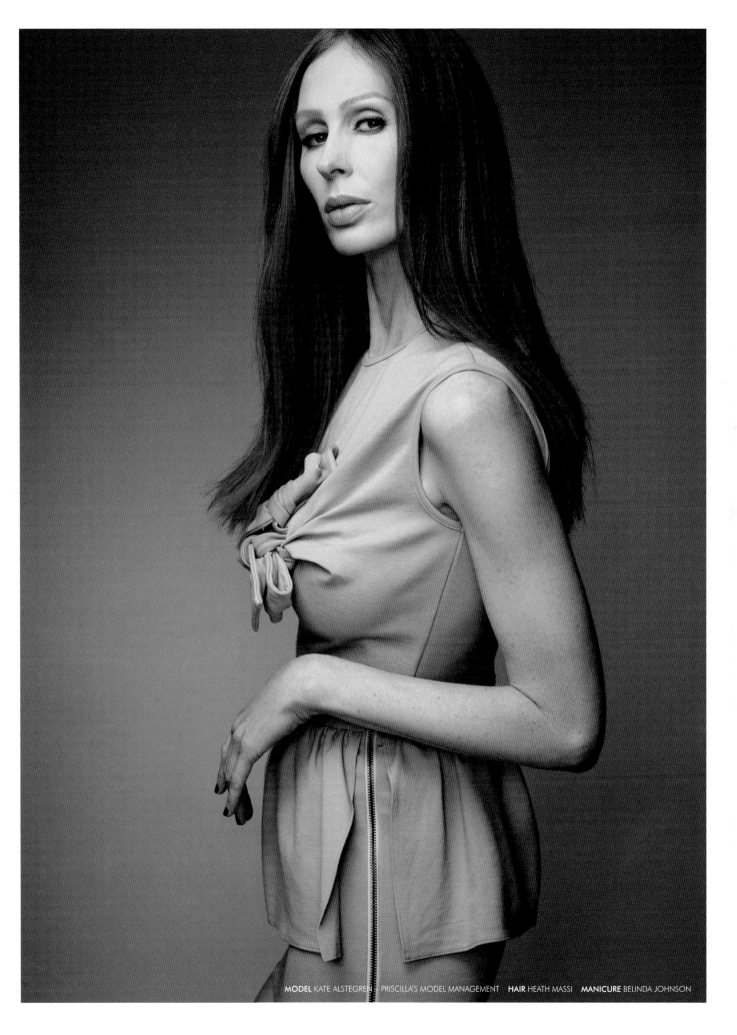

11 | EBONY RICH

A HOT BUT UTTERLY TIMELESS LOOK FOR ANY OCCASION.

1 PREP, FOUNDATION & POWDER

Prep your skin. Apply foundation, and use a matte powder to kill any shine. I love it when black/dark skins are matte, as it softens the look.

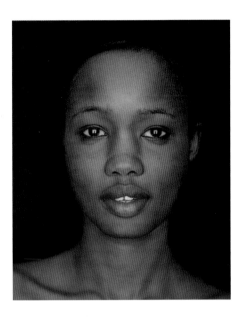

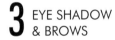

2 EYELINER & LASHES

To open up your eyes, apply a bone- or beige-coloured pencil to the inner rim of each eyelid. Apply an intense liquid black eyeliner along your top eyelids. Then curl your lashes, apply mascara and finish with false 3/4 lashes.

3 EYE SHADOW & BROWS

Use a black gel eyeliner as eye shadow. This is great for intense eyes and lasts all night. Just make sure you blend it quickly, as it dries fast. Define your brows.

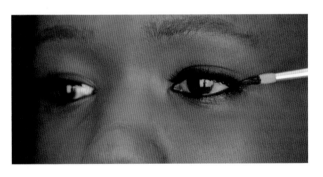

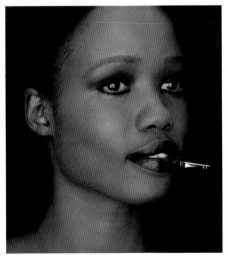

4 EYELINER & LIPS

Then apply the same black gel eyeliner underneath the bottom lash line. Finish with a burgundy-black lipstick and a deep burgundy blush.

To define your eyes, apply a few extra coats of black gel eyeliner into your eye sockets.

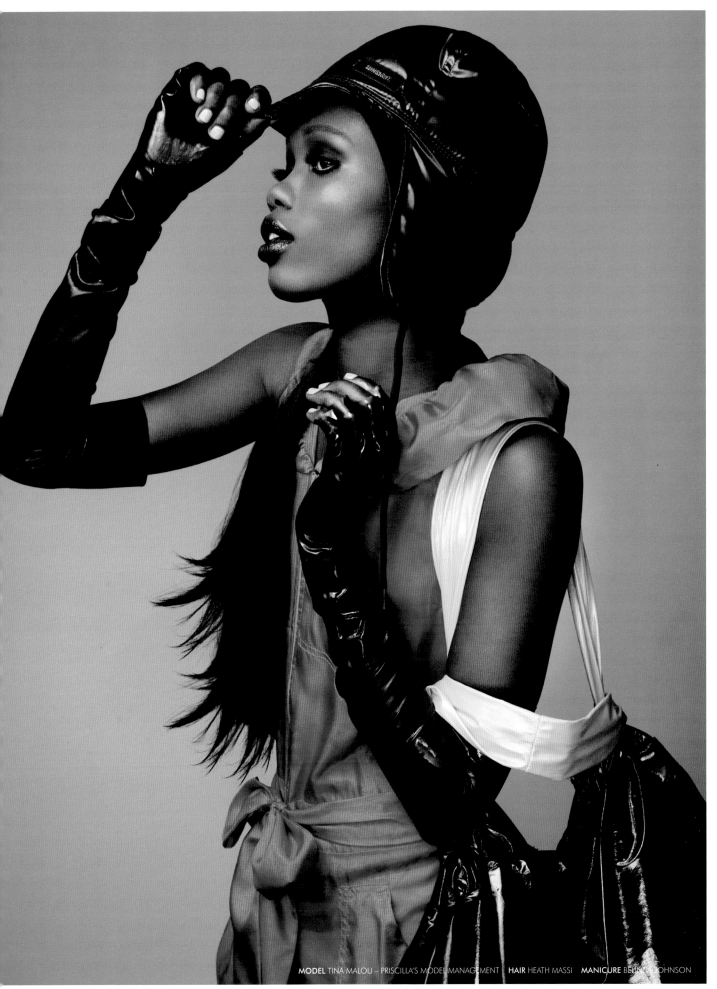

12 DUSTY CAMELLIA

SCARED OF BRIGHT
COLOURS? HERE'S
A DIVINE SOLUTION.

1 PREP &
EYELINER

All I've applied to the
model's amazing skin is
a tinted sunscreen and
a little concealer on her
eyes and around her
nostrils. Remove all the
oil from your lids and
prep them well.

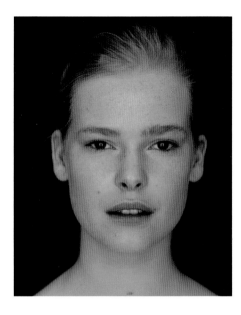

2 EYELINER

Use a chocolate-brown pencil to blend
along the entire line, then use a clean
brush to blend the pencil in a semi-
circle into your eye socket. Set this
shape with a matching matte eye
shadow and blend. This is a great
trick for flat eyelids.

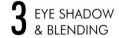

3 EYE SHADOW
& BLENDING

Do a soft wash of a reddish brown eye
shadow over your whole eyelid, again
extending it softly into your brow. Then
apply a dark brown kohl pencil on your
bottom lash line and smudge with the
same eye shadow underneath.

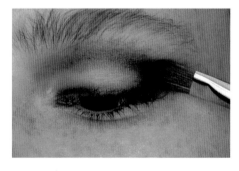

4 LASHES,
CHEEKS & LIPS

Curl your eyelashes, then apply lots of
black mascara to your top and bottom
lashes. Add a cream bronzed blush to
your cheeks. Finish off by using a matte
coral lip pencil along the whole lip,
keeping your lip beautifully matte.

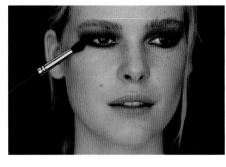

*If your lips feel a bit
dry, dab a little lip
balm on them.*

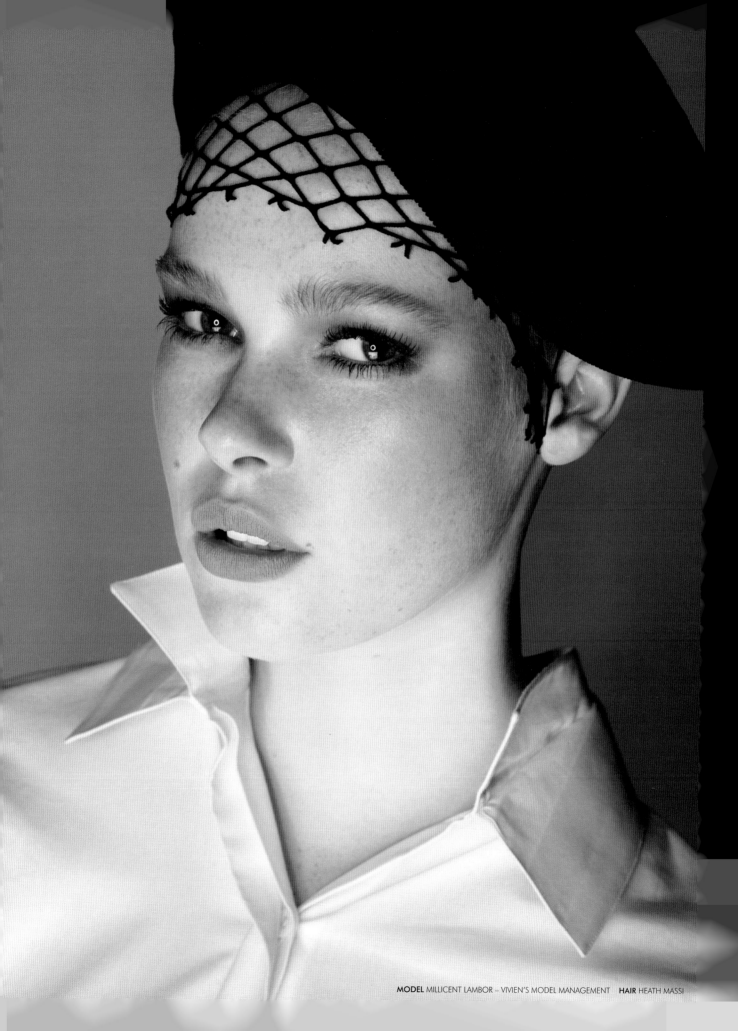

13 | SEDUCTIVE SILK

A LUMINOUS, POLISHED LOOK, PERFECT FOR DAY.

1 PREP, EYELINER & LASHES

Apply a tinted moisturiser to your face as the base, then apply a white pencil to the inner rim of each eye before curling your lashes and applying lots of black mascara to both your top and bottom lashes. Finish by applying false separated lashes.

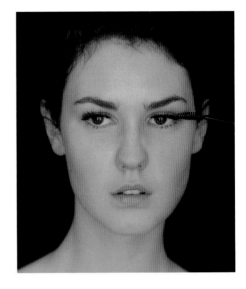

2 EYE PREP & EYE SHADOW

First, softly powder your lids for easy blending, then use a soft lavender wash of eye shadow over each eyelid.

3 CHEEKS & LIPS

Apply a soft pink blush to your cheeks and a brown lipstick to your lips.

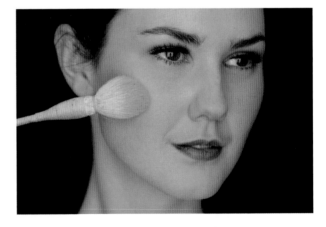

4 HIGHLIGHTER

Highlight your skin (see 'Highlight', pages 72–4).

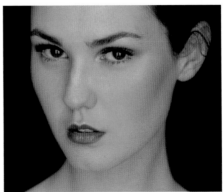

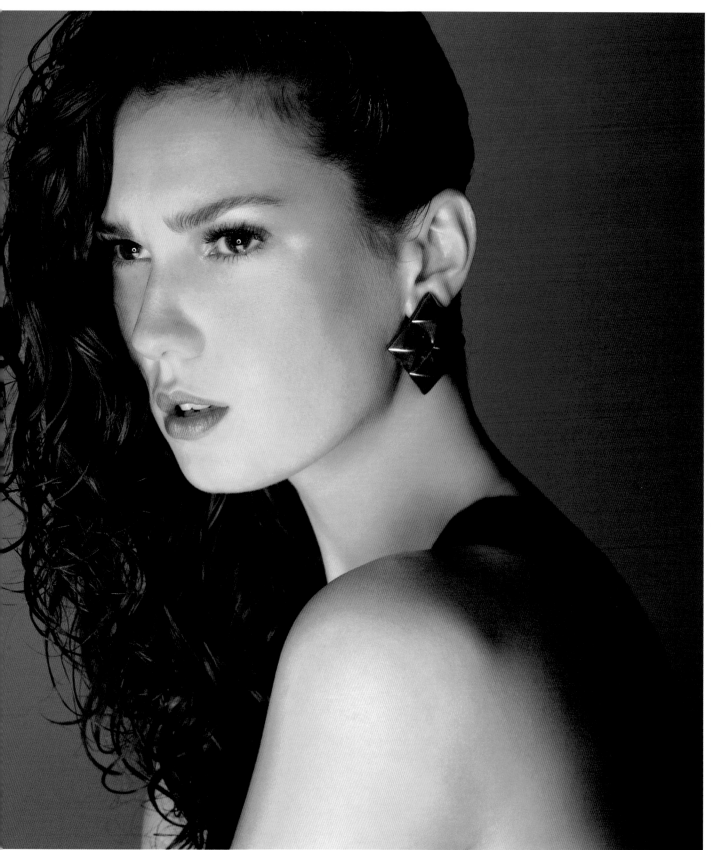

14 | KOHL GLAMOUR

AN UNDERSTATED
SULTRY LOOK FOR
WOMEN OF ALL AGES.

1 PREP & EYE SHADOW

Prep your skin, then lightly powder your lids. Apply a soft wash of matte brown eye shadow, keeping the intensity close to your eyelash line. Then, using an eye shadow brush, smudge a kohl chocolate-brown pencil along the top of each eyelash line.

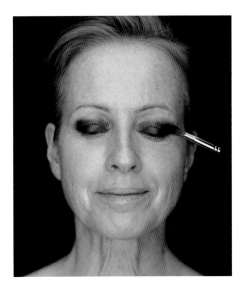

2 LOWER DEFINITION & BLENDING

Next, use a creamy white pencil on the inner rim of each eye to help conceal redness and tiredness. Apply a soft wash of matte brown eye shadow under each eye, and blend well. Finally, use chocolate-brown gel eyeliner, which is waterproof, and softly blend under the eye.

3 LASHES, BROWS & FOUNDATION

Curl your lashes and apply lots of black mascara top and bottom, then—if you're game—add some lashes. Clean away any fallout, apply a liquid foundation and define your brows. The model's eyebrows are naturally ash, so to make them look more beautiful I put brown mascara through them. When you fill in your brow, make sure you match the pencil to your brow colour.

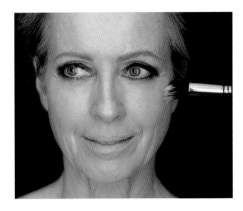

4 POWDER, CHEEKS & LIPS

Apply a soft translucent powder all over your face, then a soft peach blush and matching lip colour.

Matte colours help disguise wrinkles. It's important to do 90% of your eye makeup looking straight ahead. If there's a wrinkle or a crease, just put colour straight over it.

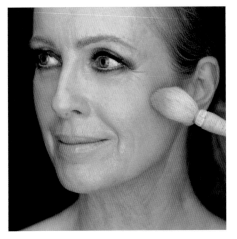

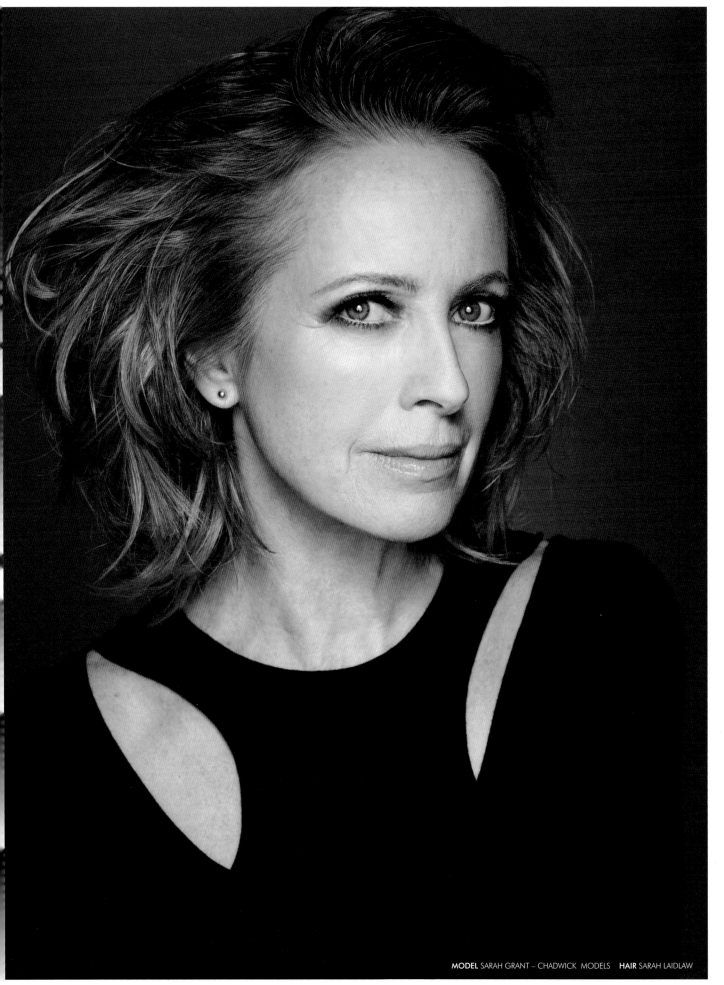

MODEL SARAH GRANT – CHADWICK MODELS **HAIR** SARAH LAIDLAW

15 NOIR CANDY

A PREPPY, FRESH LOOK THAT'S GREAT FOR ANY TIME, ANY PLACE.

1 PREP, FOUNDATION & POWDER

Prep your skin, apply foundation and then apply a matte powder all over. Define your brows, and apply a deep matte burgundy blush to your cheeks (you can also use an eye shadow for this) and blend. Clean up any fallout.

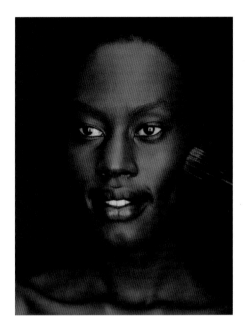

2 EYES & LIPS

Curl your lashes, then apply mascara to your top and bottom lashes. Add false separated lashes. Run a black liquid eyeliner along the top and bottom of each eyelid. Finally, apply a deep burgundy lipstick.

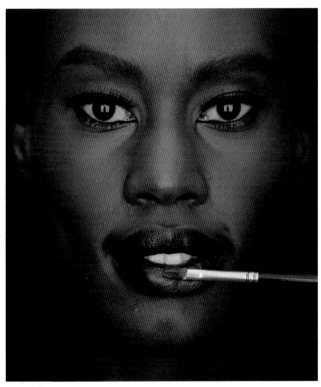

Because the model's brows are naturally so arched, I brought the arch down to give her a more sophisticated look.

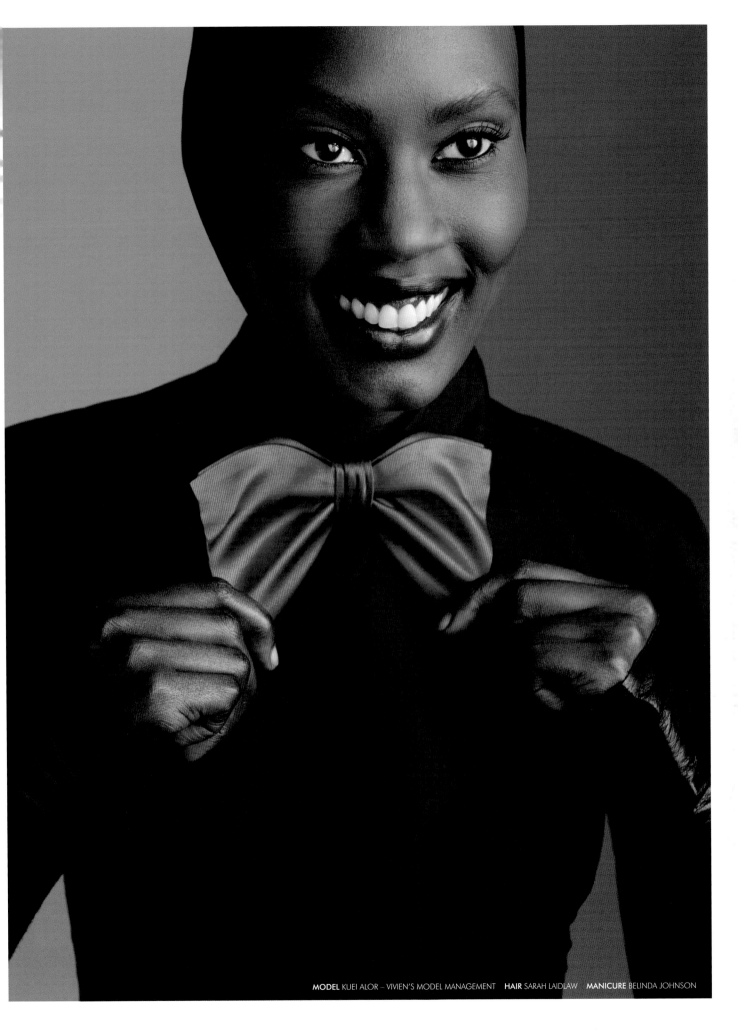

16 | NATURALLY SUMPTUOUS

A SOFT BUT GROOMED
AND ELEGANT LOOK.

1 LASHES

First, curl your lashes,
then apply thick mascara
to both your top and
bottom lashes. Next,
add false 3/4 lashes to
your top lashes only.

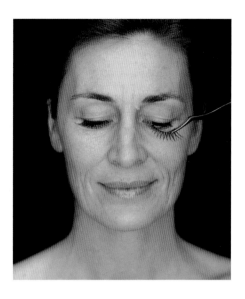

2 SKIN PREP & BROWS

Lightly apply a liquid foundation, and concealer where
it's needed, then use a translucent powder all over your
face. Define your eyebrows with an angle brush, and
you'll see what a difference groomed brows make.

3 CHEEKS & EYELIDS

Use a kabuki brush to apply a soft coral
blush high on your cheekbones. Lightly
wash this colour over your eyelids, then
choose your correct highlighter shade
and highlight your cupid's bow and the
inner corners of your eyes. Apply a soft
berry-pink lipstick.

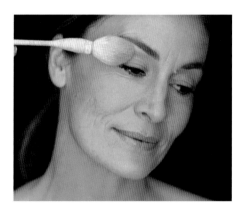

*Don't smile when you
apply blush, otherwise
you'll cause lines.*

4 EYELINER & PENCIL

Softly apply a brown-
black gel eyeliner under
your bottom lash line,
then a creamy white
pencil to the inner rims
of each eye before blend-
ing it until it looks soft
and smudged.

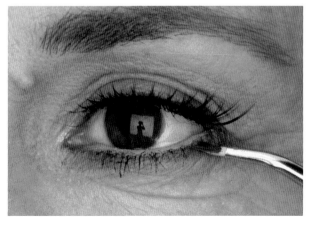

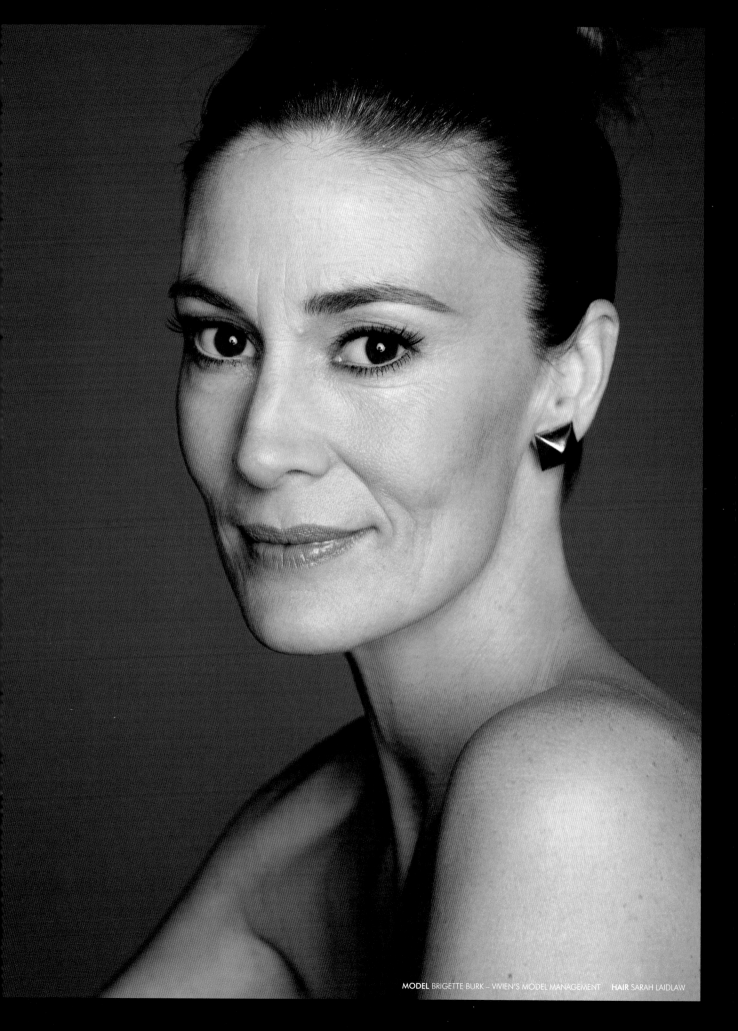

17 | ESPECIALLY CITRUS

GLITTERING EYE MAKEUP
IS SIMPLE TO APPLY BUT
ALWAYS STUNNING.

1 GLITTER EYE SHADOW

Put cream under your
eyes to help catch the
fallout, then apply a light
wash of latex/eyelash
glue to your lids. When
it's sticky, tilt your head
back and look into the
mirror. Pat the glitter
onto each lid with your
fingertip and blend.
Clean up the cream and
any fallout, then apply a
liquid foundation before
lightly powdering.

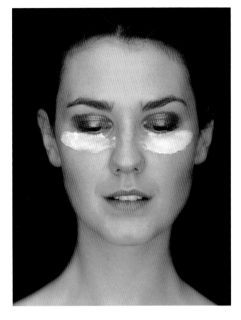

2 EYELINER & EYE SHADOW

Take a black gel eyeliner and wipe any
excess from the applicator on the back
of your hand. Smudge the eyeliner
into your natural socket line. A good
blending trick is to use a matte soft
eye shadow on a clean brush. Next,
groom your eyebrows and apply lots
of mascara to your top lashes only.

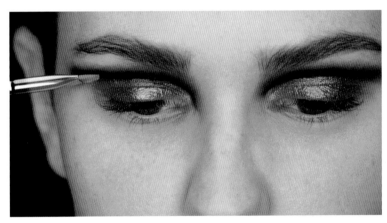

3 LASHES

After you've cleaned
up any fallout, apply
foundation and, if
necessary, concealer.
Finish with a berry lip-
stick and matching blush.

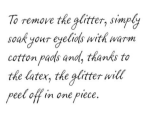

*To remove the glitter, simply
soak your eyelids with warm
cotton pads and, thanks to
the latex, the glitter will
peel off in one piece.*

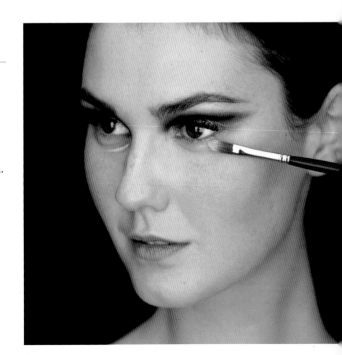

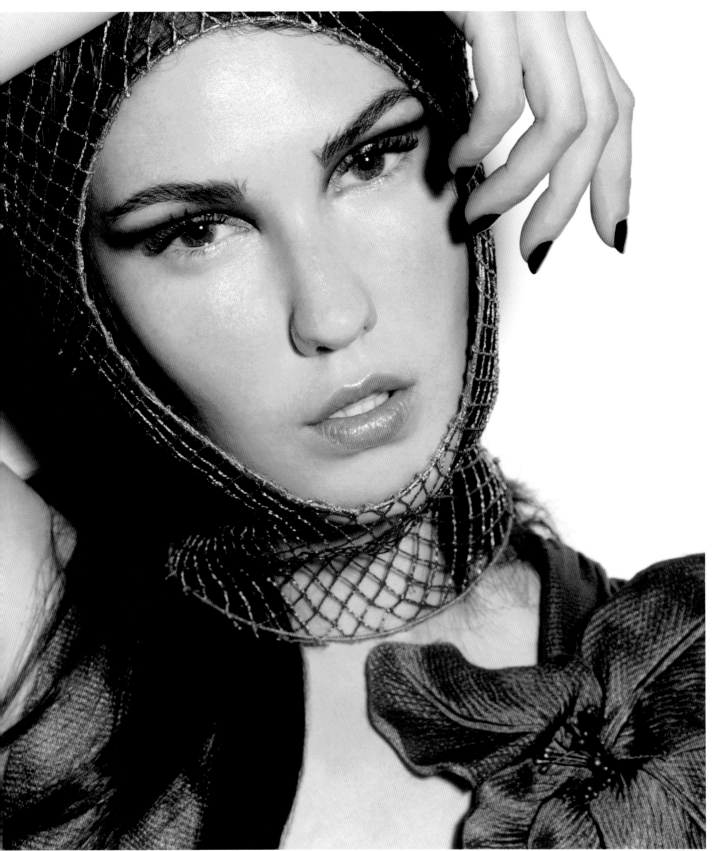

MODEL RACHAEL GRASSO – VIVIEN'S MODEL MANAGEMENT **HAIR** SARAH LAIDLAW **MANICURE** BELINDA JOHNSON

18 | ATOMIC ORANGE

LIVEN UP BROWN SHADES
WITH INTENSE ORANGE.

1 EYE SHADOW

Prep your eyelids and
apply a shimmery bronze
eye shadow to your entire
lids. Don't worry about
any fallout, as you can
clean it up later. Use a
soft bronze eye shadow
to blend it up to each
brow bone, just under
your eyebrow.

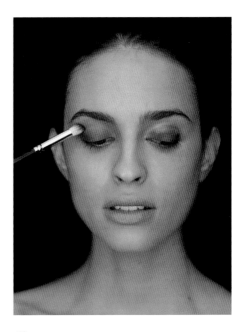

2 EYELINER

Wet a fine angle brush
and use it to apply an
intense orange pigment
as an eyeliner along each
top eyelash line.

*The best nudes are the colours between your natural lip colour
and your natural skin colour. If you use a lipstick that's the
same colour as your foundation, you'll look as if you have no lips.*

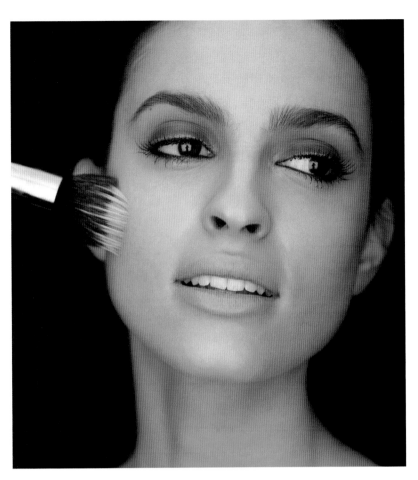

3 EYES, FOUNDATION & HIGHLIGHTER

Curl your lashes, and apply lots of mascara to both your top and bottom lashes. Apply a chocolate kohl eye pencil to the inner rim of each eye. Clean up any fallout and apply liquid foundation. Highlight your skin if you wish (see pages 72–4).

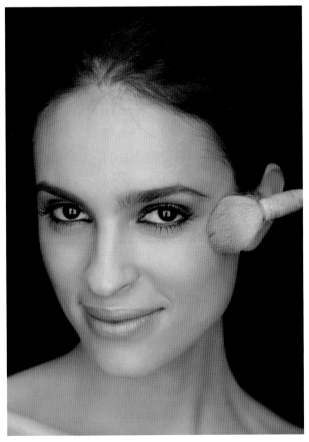

4 CHEEKS & LIPS

Apply a really soft cream burgundy blush to your cheeks, then use your finger to slightly stain your lip with the same blush. Next, apply a cream apricot blush to your cheeks. Finally, highlight your lips and apply a soft nude lipstick.

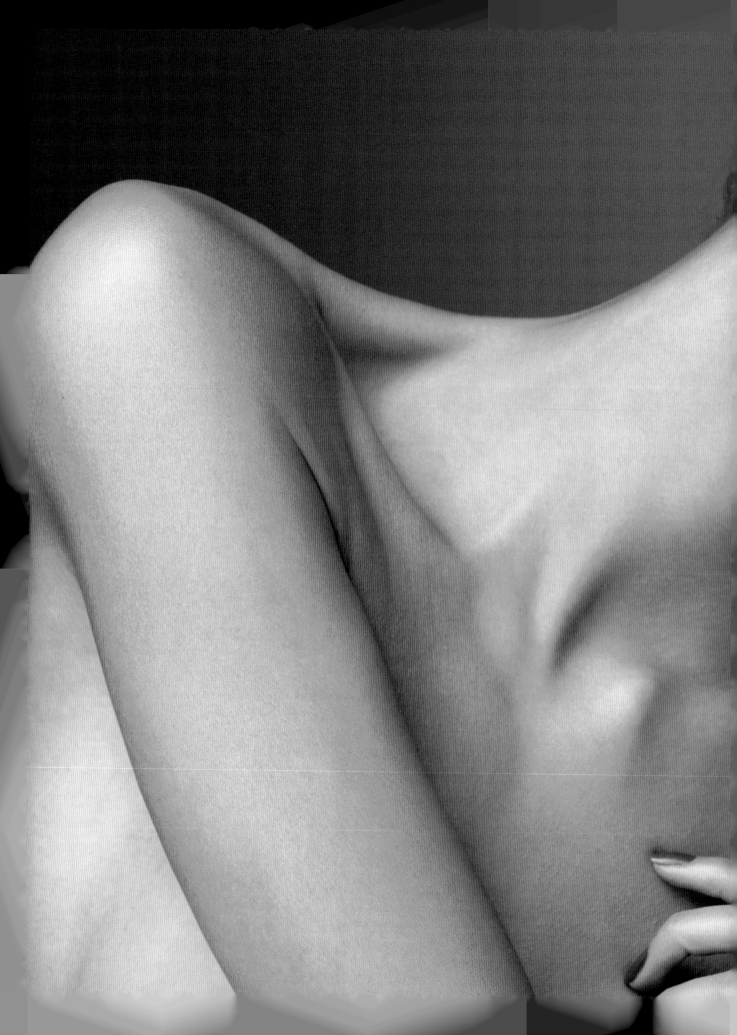

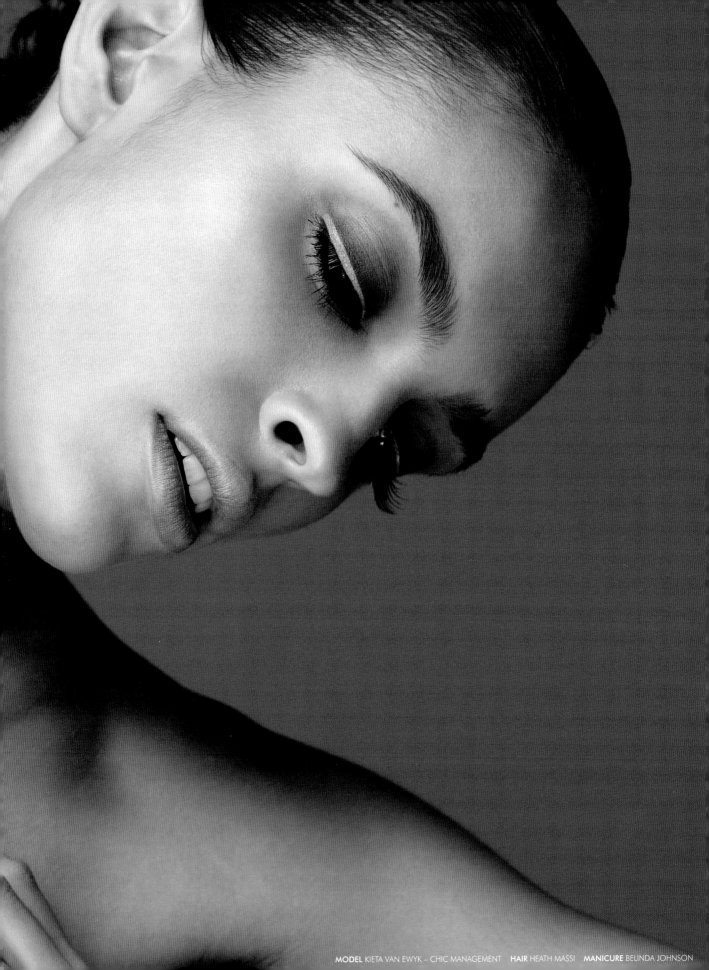

19 | KILLER ONYX

AN EASY-TO-APPLY
GRAPHIC EYE THAT
WILL LAST ALL NIGHT.

1 EYE SHADOW

Prep your eyes. Following the natural contour of your eyes, apply sticky tape, then lightly brush matte deep purple eye shadow along your lash lines up onto the tape (for detailed instructions, see page 94).

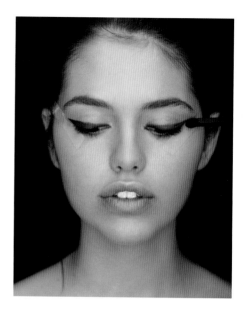

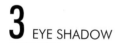

2 EYELINER

Remove the tape, then apply black kohl pencil to the inner rim of each eye. Smudge into the outer corners of each top lash line.

3 EYE SHADOW

Blend a black eye shadow along your bottom lash lines. If you're having trouble blending, use some translucent powder on a clean brush. Clean up any fallout and apply a cream foundation.

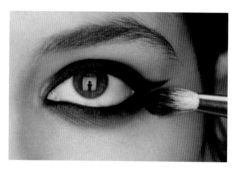

The inner rim pencil has a tendency to fade, so you may need to reapply this throughout the day or night.

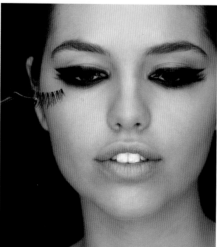

4 LASHES, CHEEKS & LIPS

Curl your lashes, then apply lots of black mascara to your top and bottom lashes. Apply false wispy lashes. Finally, lightly contour your cheeks, and apply a clear lip balm to your lips.

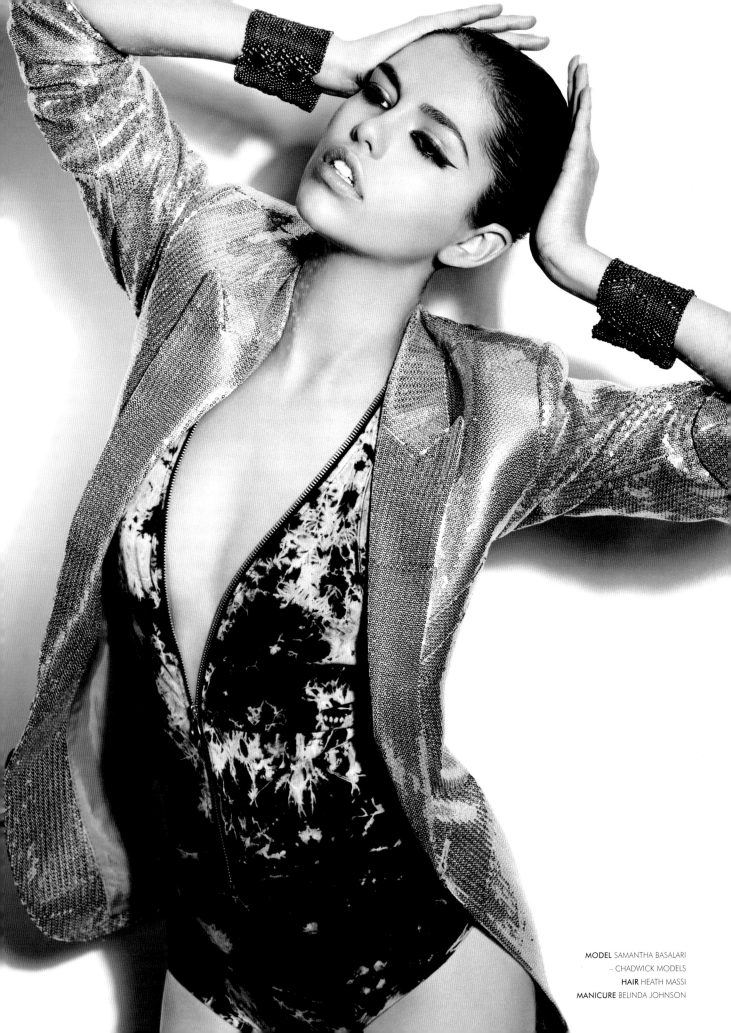

MODEL SAMANTHA BASALARI
– CHADWICK MODELS
HAIR HEATH MASSI
MANICURE BELINDA JOHNSON

20 CRANBERRY KISS

A CLASSIC FEMININE
LOOK THAT NEVER DATES.

1 EYES, PREP & LIPS

Curl your eyelashes.
Apply black mascara,
cream foundation and
then bright red lip pencil
all over your lips.

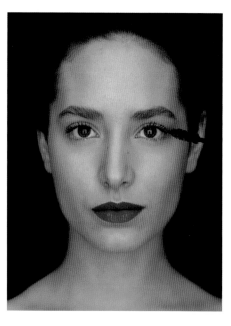

2 EYES, CHEEKS & BROWS

Apply creamy white
pencil to the inner rim
of each eye, and define
your brows. Apply a
soft bronze blush. If
you have time, apply
false 3/4 lashes.

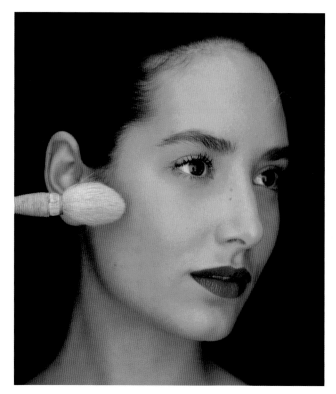

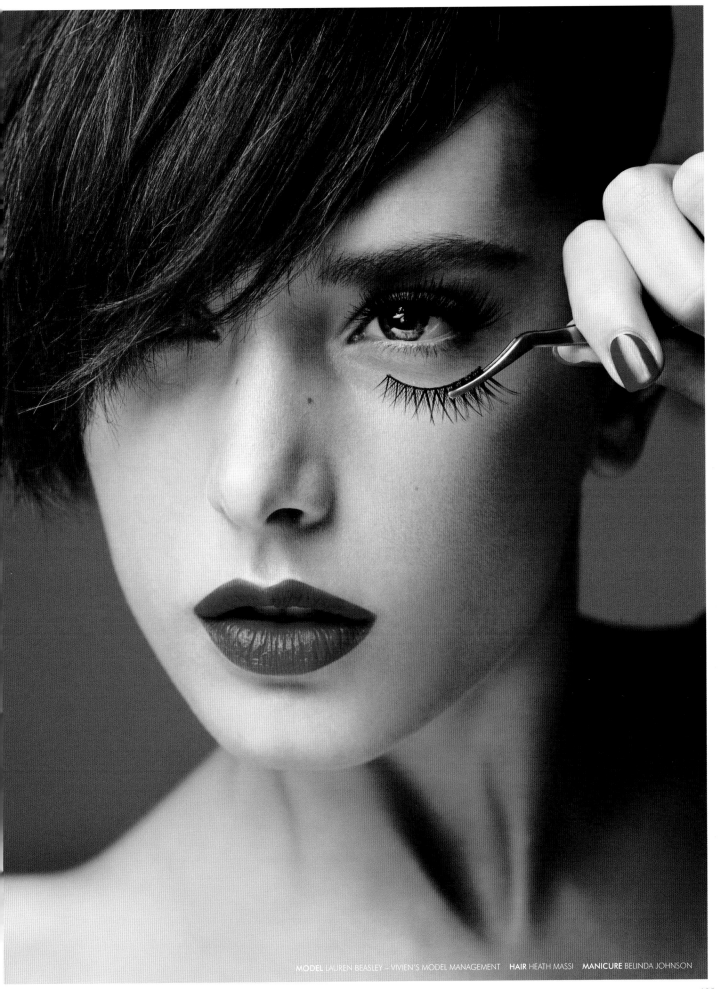

21 | ULTRA LUX

A LUXURIOUS LOOK FOR A GLAMOROUS RED CARPET EVENT.

1 PREP, FOUNDATION & POWDER

Prep your skin. Apply foundation and concealer, then lightly powder your face. This will give your skin a velvety texture. Apply soft beige nude lipstick to your lips.

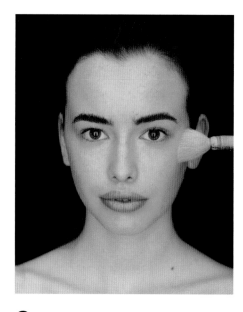

2 EYELINER

Smudge a reddish brown kohl pencil along your lash lines, then blend it with a clean brush.

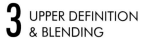

3 UPPER DEFINITION & BLENDING

Colour in your whole eyelid with an intense black kohl pencil, then take a medium-sized brush and blend, blend, blend. Repeat for the other eye.

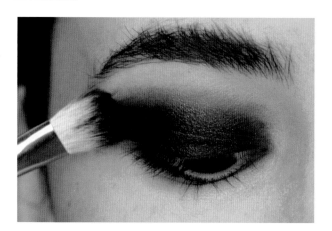

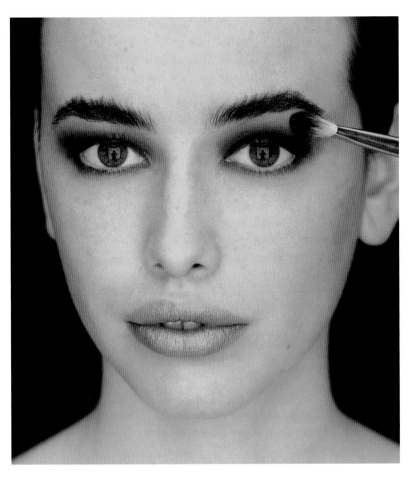

4 EYE SHADOW & BLENDING

Looking straight ahead, use a burgundy-red eye shadow to blend the black closer to your eyebrows.

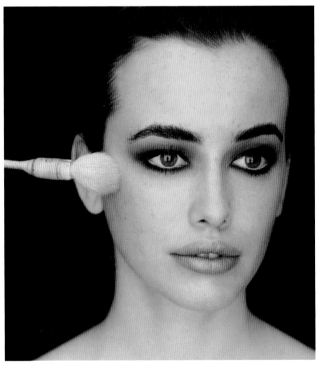

5 LASHES, CHEEKS & BROWS

Smudge more black kohl pencil into your bottom lash lines. Curl your lashes, then apply lots of mascara to your top and bottom lashes. Add false 3/4 lashes. Finish off with a soft peach blush and, finally, define your brows.

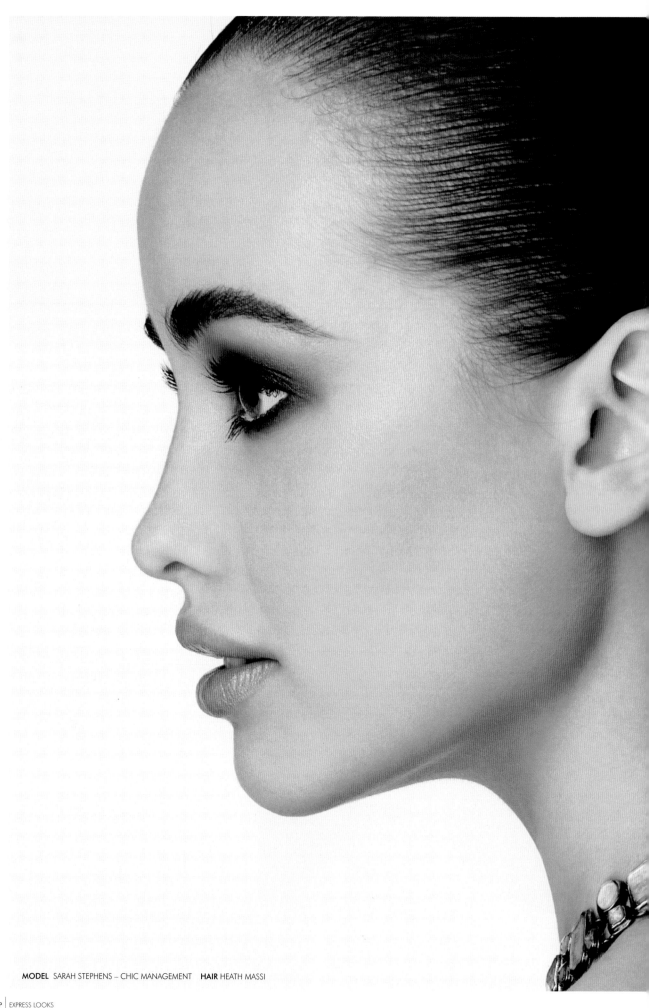

MODEL SARAH STEPHENS – CHIC MANAGEMENT **HAIR** HEATH MASSI

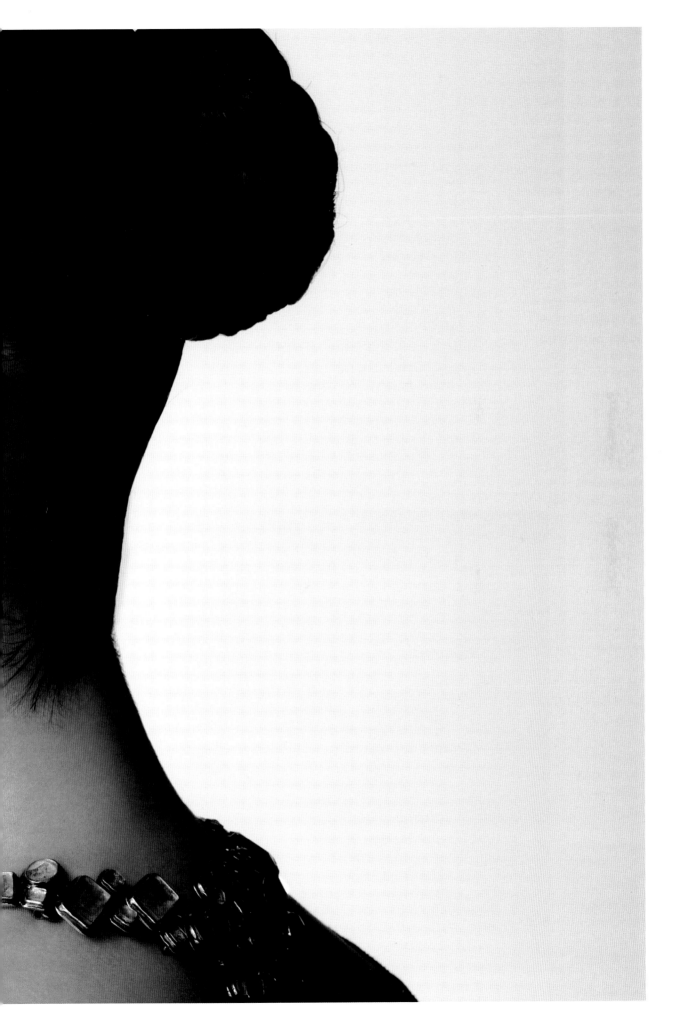

22 | GOLDEN MAGNOLIA

REJUVENATE TIRED SKIN
WITH A HOLIDAY GLOW.

1 PREP & EYES

Prep your skin before
applying cream liquid
foundation. Then apply
a gold shimmer pigment
with a wet brush. With
the same gold colour,
highlight your skin. Take
a bronze kohl eye pencil
and smudge along your
top eyelash lines. Use an
angled brush to slightly
extend the line outwards.

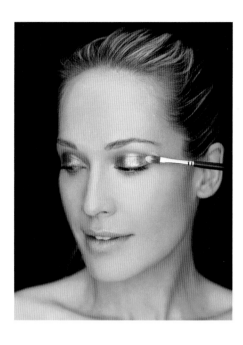

2 LASHES & LIPS

Apply a creamy white
pencil to the inner rims
of your eyes. Curl your
lashes, then apply lots
of mascara to your top
lashes only. Finish by
applying a rose-tinted
cream blush to your
cheeks and lips. You
can add a clear gloss
if you wish.

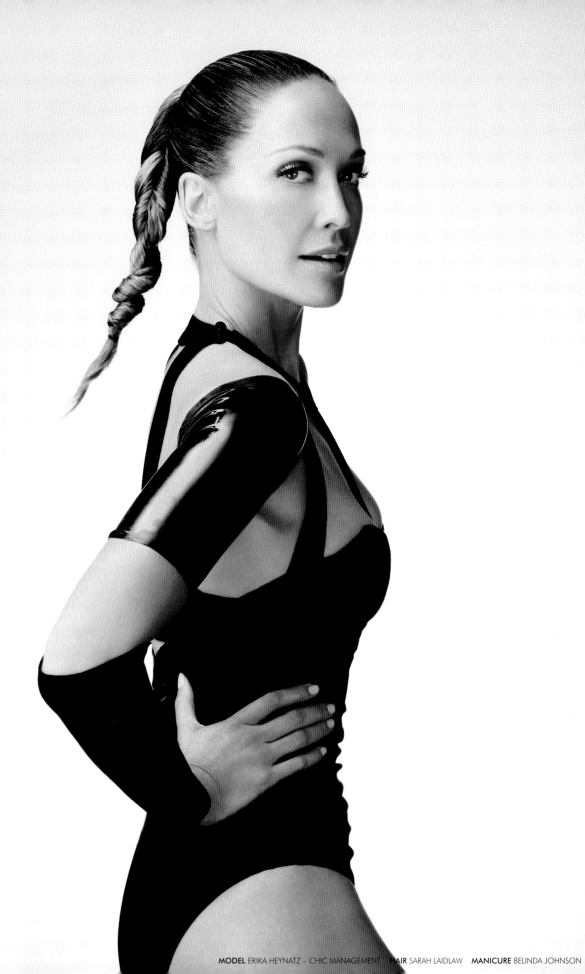

23 | VIVA RADIANCE

A QUICK WAY TO LIFT
YOUR EYES AND LOOK
YEARS YOUNGER.

1 FOUNDATION & CHEEKS

Give yourself a healthy
glow by using a rich
creamy foundation
before applying a cream
concealer under your
eyes. Then apply a rose-
coloured cream blush
high on your cheeks.
Remember not to smile,
or you'll cause wrinkles.

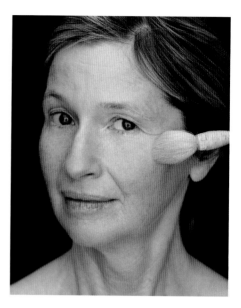

2 BROWS, EYE PREP & LASHES

Define your brows with a
brow pencil that matches
your brow hair colour.
Powder your lids with
translucent powder.
Remember, 99% of your eye
shadow is going to be done
looking straight ahead (see
step 3). Curl your lashes.

3 EYE SHADOW

Looking straight into the mirror, colour
in your eyelids with a matte soft grey
eye shadow, as shown, then look down
so you can fill in any gaps you may have
missed. Don't worry about any fallout,
which you can clean up later.

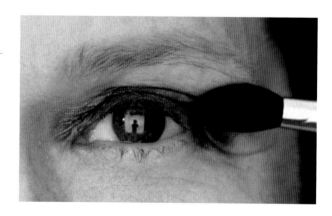

*Never wear a frosty eye shadow or lipstick,
as it will age you ten years in an instant.*

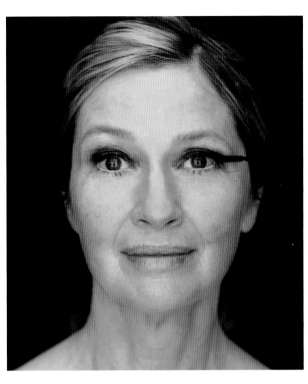

4 LASHES & INNER RIMS

Clean up any fallout with a baby wipe, then use concealer under your eyes. Apply lots of black mascara, adding more to your top lashes. Apply creamy white pencil to the inner rim of each eye.

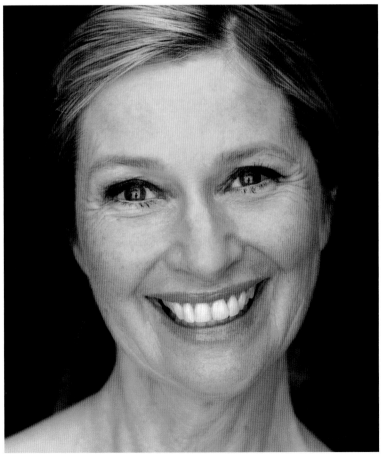

5 CHEEKS & LIPS

If necessary, apply more blush, as it has a tendency to blend into the skin. Use a soft nude lipstick that is closest to your natural lip colour. If your skin is oily or becomes shiny easily, this is a great time to blot it with either a tissue or non-powdered blotting paper before applying light powder. If your skin is dry, however, don't use powder.

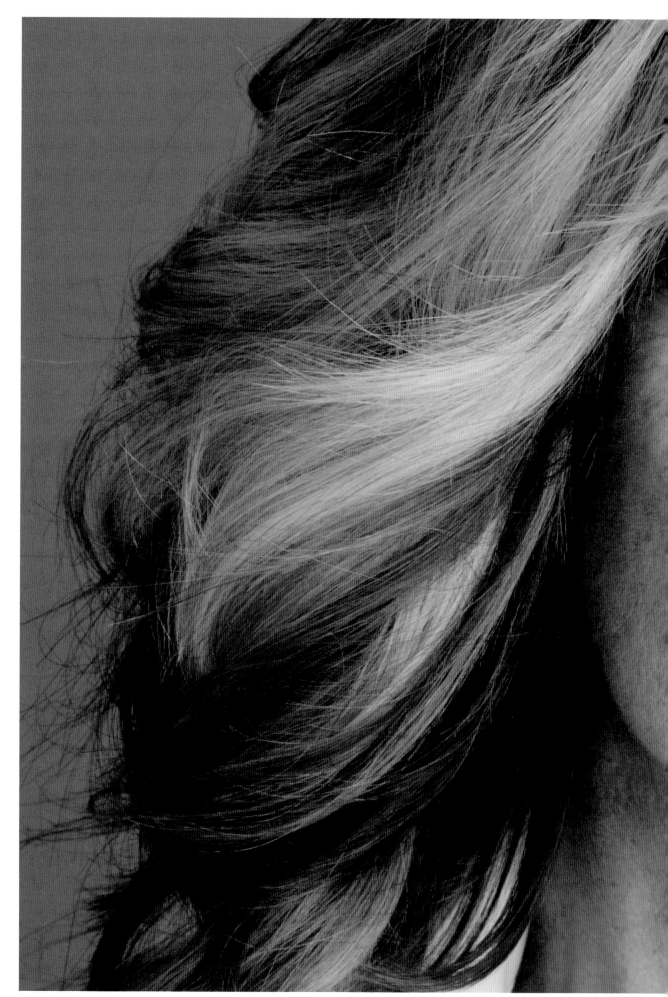

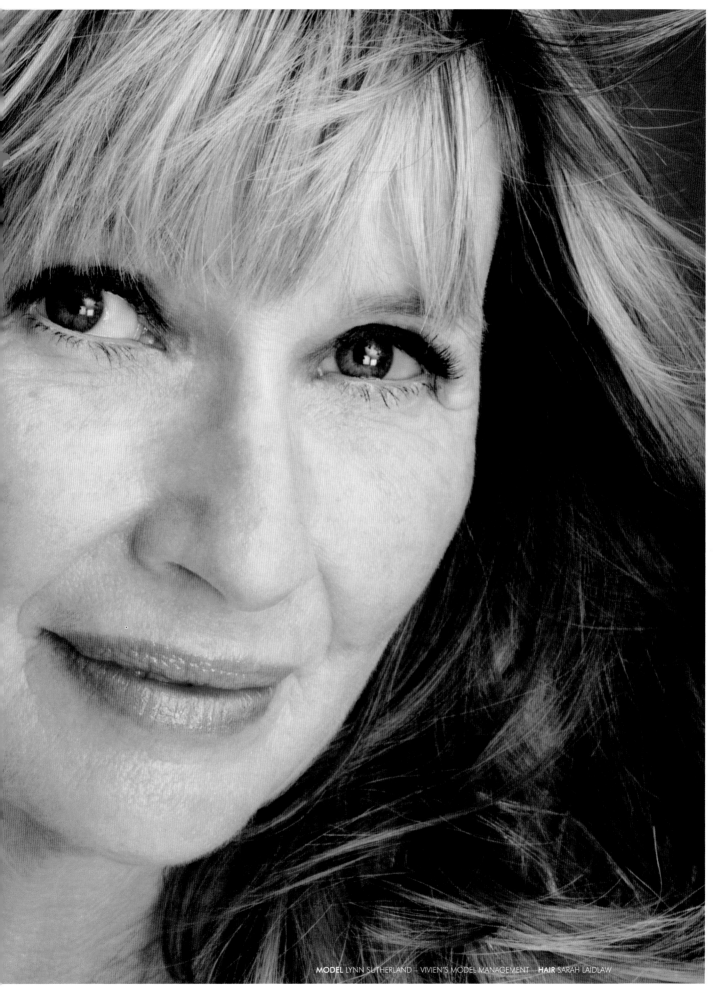

24 | ALLURING PERFECTION

GRACEFUL ELEGANCE WITH
A SOFT MAHOGANY EYE.

1 EYE PREP & BROWS

Prep your eyelids.
Use concealer where
necessary, and define
your brows with an
angle brush so that you
get full, feathery brows.

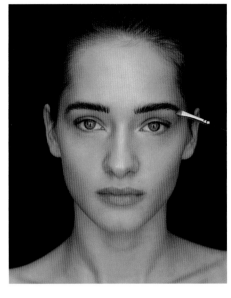

2 LASHES & EYELINER

Curl your lashes, and apply
lots of mascara to your top
lashes only. Using an angle
brush, press a black gel
eyeliner into the lashes
on your top lash lines.

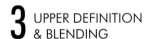

3 UPPER DEFINITION & BLENDING

Looking straight ahead into the mirror, use
a mahogany-brown eye shadow to follow
the natural shape of your brow bones and
extend out. Remember to blend well.

*For this look I've applied a few single eyelashes.
You can do this too, if you have time. Don't worry
if the eyelash glue is white, as it dries clear.*

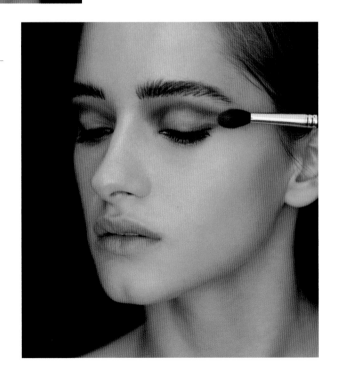

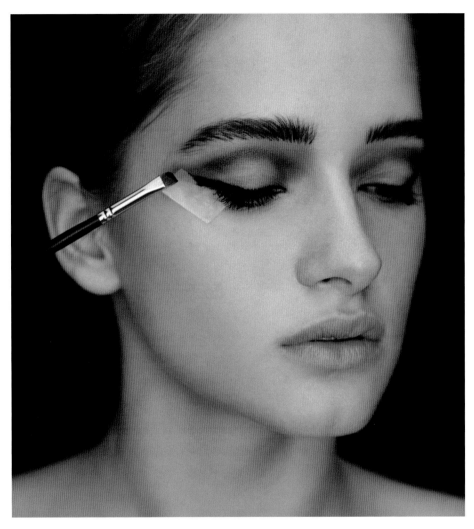

4 POWDER & KOHL PENCIL

To intensify this look, use liquid black eyeliner and some sticky tape to create a strong black line (see page 94). Peel the tape off. Remove any extra sheen from your face with non-powdered blotting paper, then add a dusting of powder. Generously apply brown kohl pencil to the inner rims of your eyes.

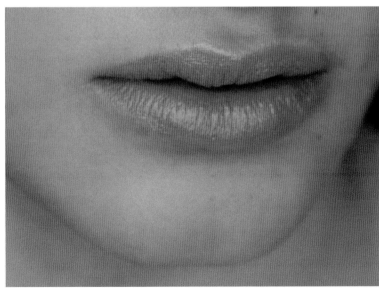

5 LIPS & CHEEKS

Apply a hint of lip balm. If your lips don't have as much natural colour as the model's, add just a hint of deep berry- or plum-coloured lip stain. Also add a small amount of cream blush.

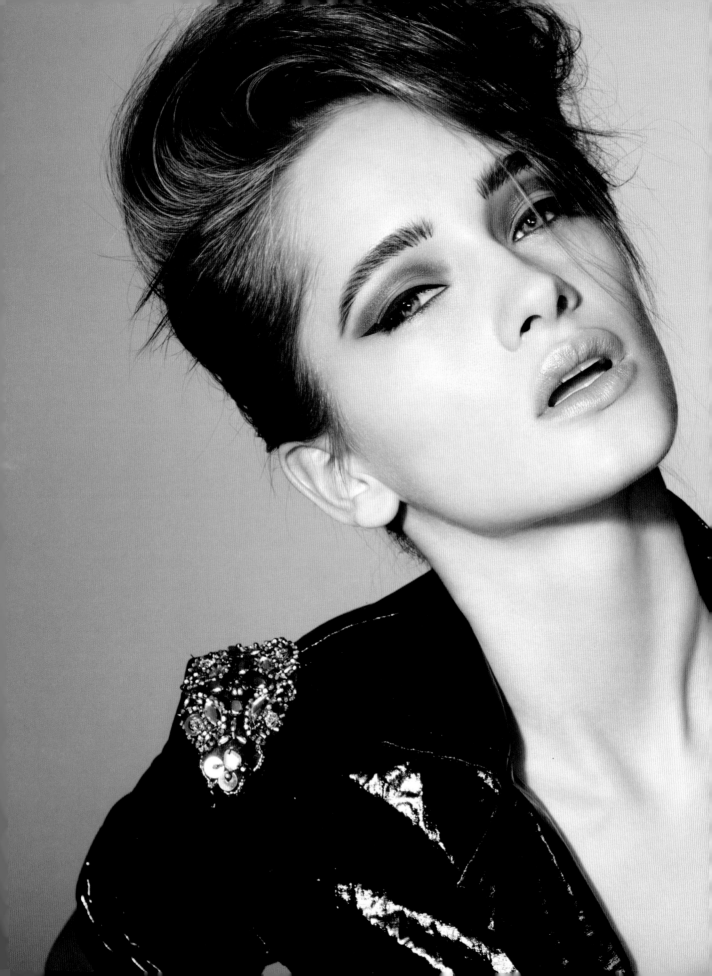

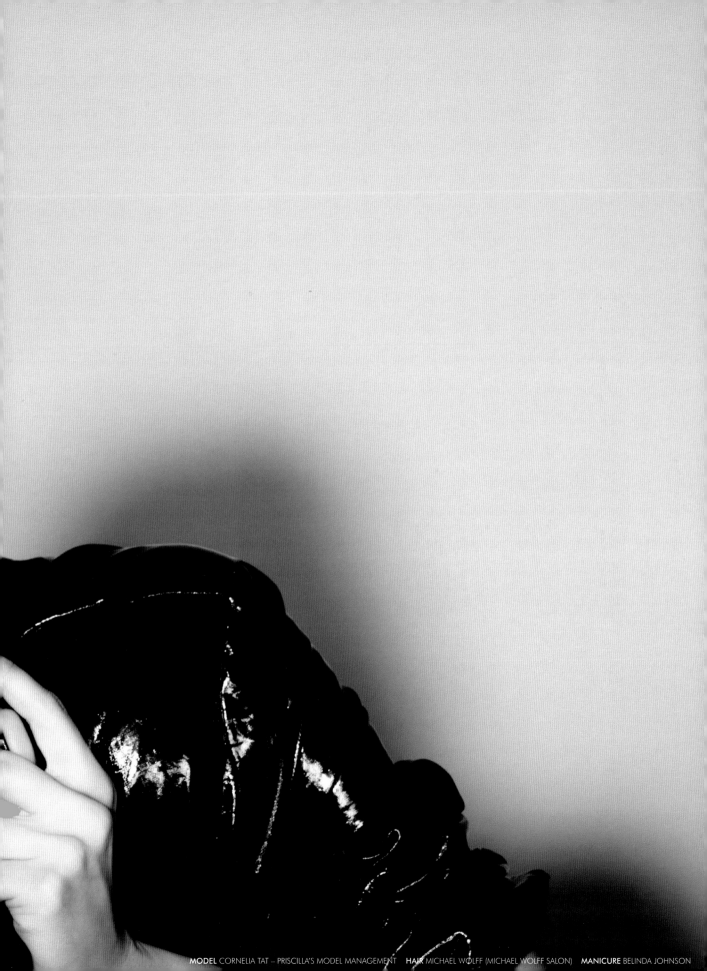

25 | NEON VOGUE

AN INTENSE CATWALK
LOOK FOR EVENING.

1 EYE PREP & PIGMENT

Put a wash of liquid foundation on your eyelids. Don't apply any powder, as the pigment needs to stick. Put some cream under your eyes to catch any fallout, then apply an intense orange pigment to your eyelids.

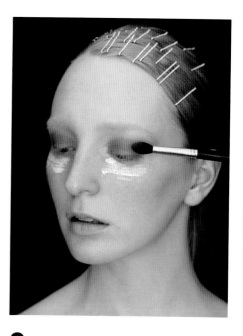

2 UPPER DEFINITION & LASHES

Take a strong violet eye shadow and blend along your natural socket line. Smudge a chocolate-brown kohl pencil along your bottom eyelash line. Apply lots of mascara top and bottom.

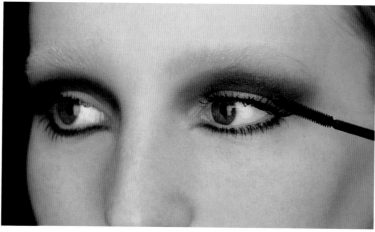

3 FOUNDATION, CHEEKS & LIPS

Apply foundation, if required. If your cheeks are naturally pink, you don't need to add blush. Finish off with strong red lips.

A very pale brow keeps the focus on the eye.

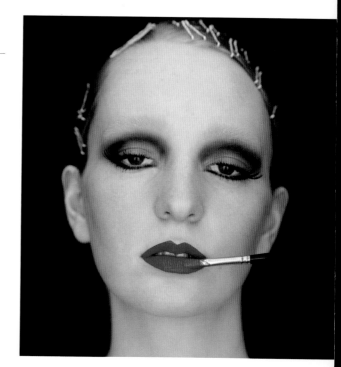

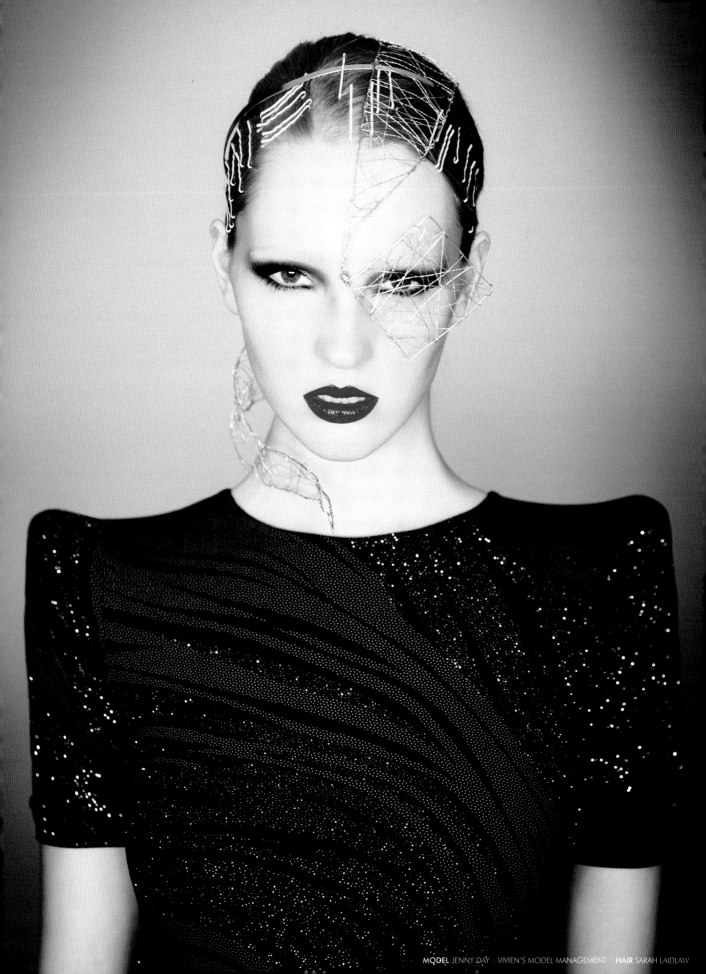

26 | TRÈS CHIC

A SOPHISTICATED LOOK
FOR STYLISH CITY GIRLS.

1 SKIN & EYE PREP

Prep your skin, then apply foundation and concealer, where required. Powder your eyelids. Do a wash of matte taupe eye shadow across your eyelids.

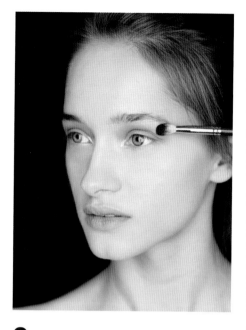

2 INNER RIMS & LASHES

Wet a fine angle brush and apply an intense silver pigment to the inner corners of your eyes. Curl your lashes, then apply lots of mascara to your top and bottom lashes.

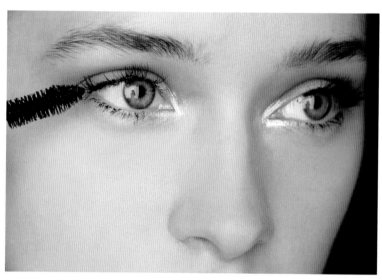

3 BROWS, CHEEKS & LIPS

Define your brows. Apply a soft rose-coloured powdered blush. Using your fingertip, and keeping it very soft and sheer, stain your lip with a deep berry- or plum-coloured lipstick.

If you never powder your face, make sure you use a cream blush for better blending.

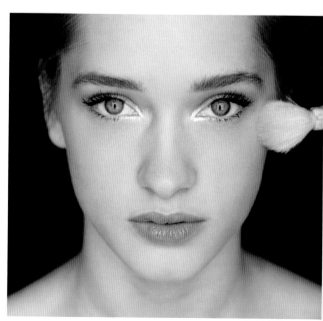

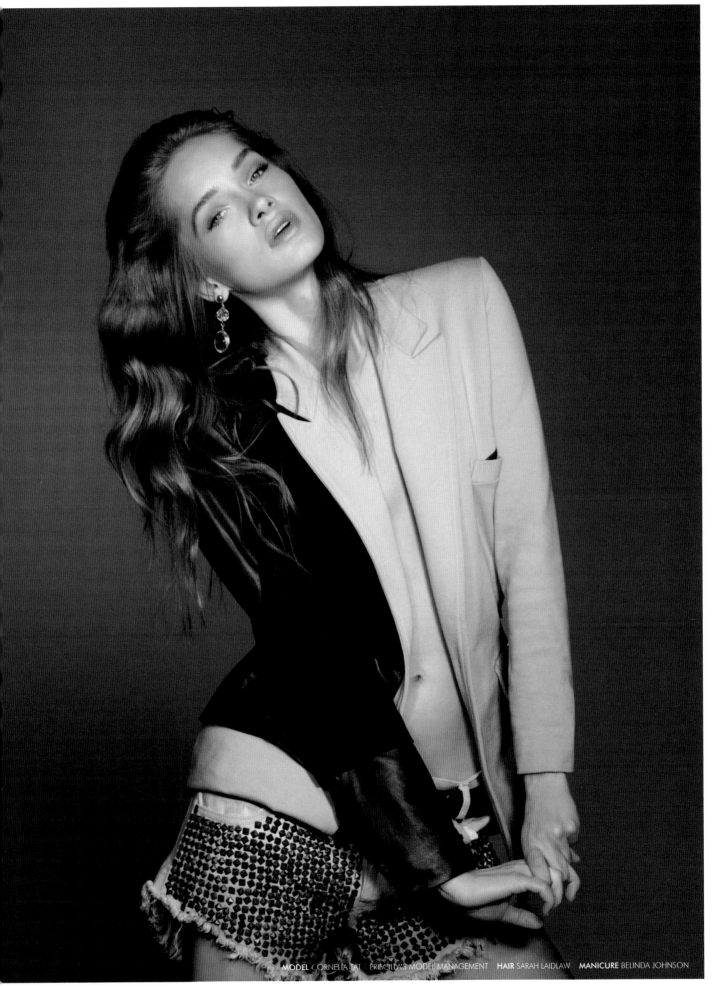

MODEL CORNELIA TAT · PRISCILLA'S MODEL MANAGEMENT **HAIR** SARAH LAIDLAW **MANICURE** BELINDA JOHNSON

27 | AMETHYST SUPREME

FLATTER BROWN EYES WITH
AUBERGINE SHADOW.

1 DEFINITION & BLENDING

Apply a deep aubergine kohl pencil to your entire eyelid, keeping all the intensity at your lash line. Do the same for the other eye. Apply the same pencil along your inner lower rims. Make sure you blend each eyelid evenly before using a matching eye shadow to blend the edges smoothly.

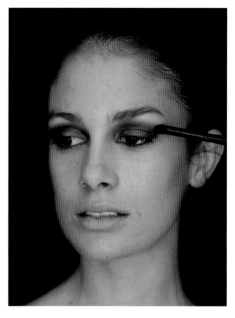

2 LASHES & EYELINER

Curl your lashes, and apply heavy mascara to your top lashes only. Then line your top lash lines with a deep violet liquid eyeliner.

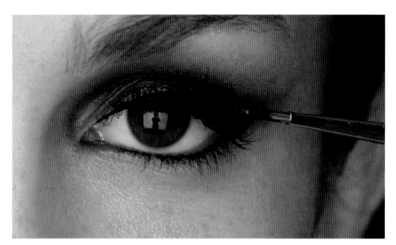

3 BROWS, CHEEKS & LIPS

Clean up any fallout, then apply foundation, or just a bit of concealer if you have great skin. Define your brows, and apply a little deep berry- or plum-coloured lip stain to your cheeks and lips. If your lips are slightly dry, add a hint of clear lip gloss. Highlight your skin if you wish.

If you have a protruding brow bone, then darken that area.

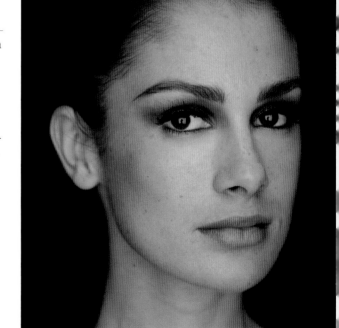

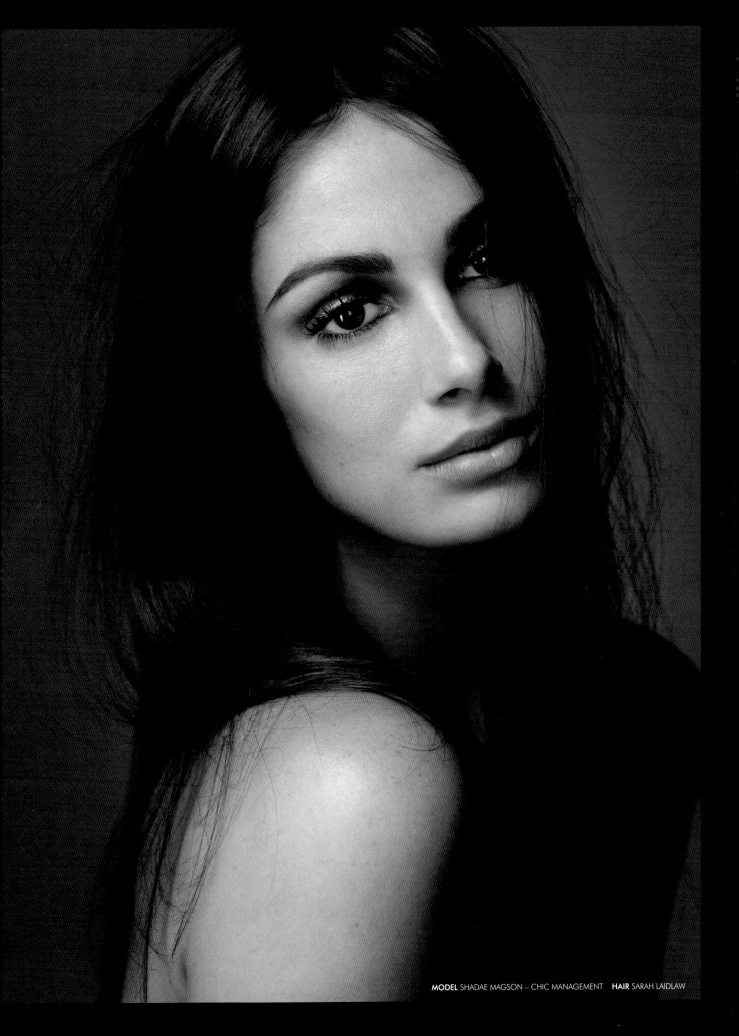

MODEL SHADAE MAGSON – CHIC MANAGEMENT   HAIR SARAH LAIDLAW

28 FIERCE FELINE

WANT TO STAND OUT?
THIS ONE'S NOT FOR
THE FAINTHEARTED.

1 EYE PREP & DEFINITION

If you want a powerful
eye look, this is the one.
Prep your eyelids first.
Apply a matte white eye
shadow to your lids. Use
a fine angle brush with a
gel eyeliner to run a thin
line along your bottom
lash lines, smudging it
into a fine point at the
inner corners.

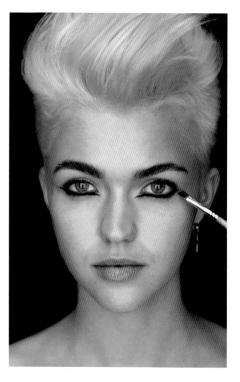

2 UPPER DEFINITION

Heavily smudge a black
kohl pencil to the outer
socket of each eyelid.
Let it heat up on your
skin for a few seconds
before smudging it
across your brow bone.

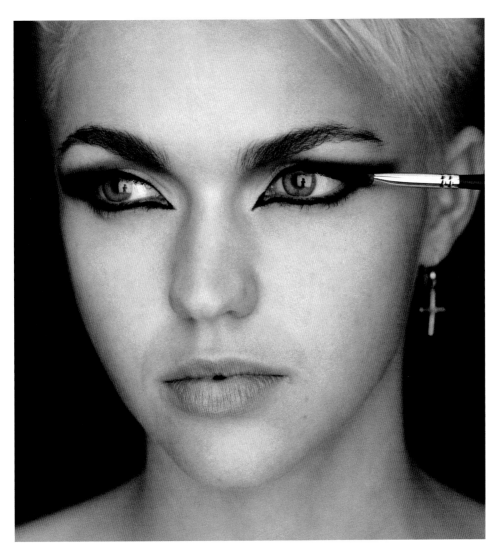

3 EYELINER

Apply an intense liquid liner along each top lash line and join it to the lower eyeliner to create a point.

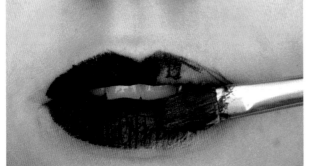

4 LASHES, BROWS & LIPS

Curl your lashes, then apply heavy mascara to the top lashes only. Use a dark pencil to both lower and strengthen each eyebrow. Use foundation only where required, then apply a black lipstick.

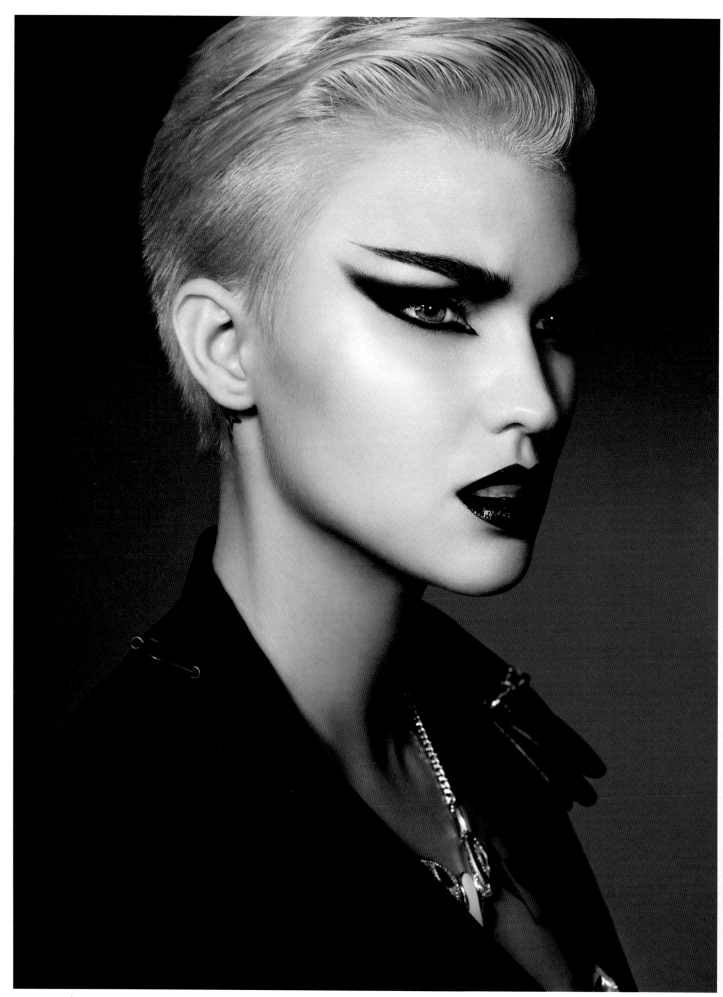

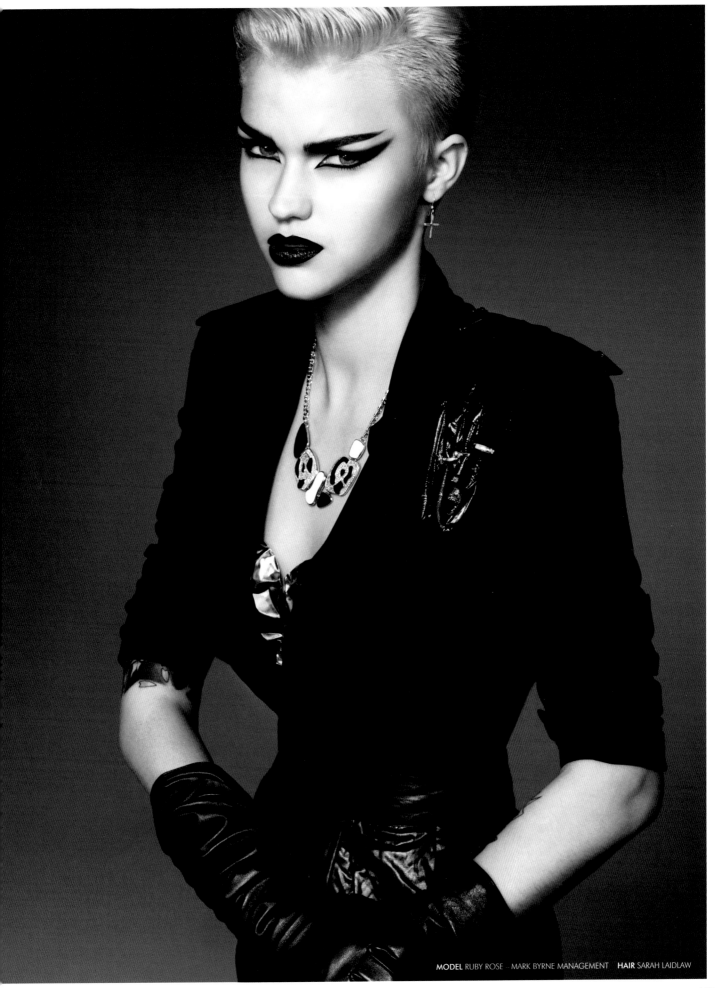

29 | SAPPHIRE BEAUTY

TRANSFORM YOUR EYES
INTO LUMINOUS POOLS.

1 EYE PREP & PIGMENT

Prep your eyelids, but don't powder them. Apply an intense blue pigment to your eyelids, then define the edges with a cotton bud.

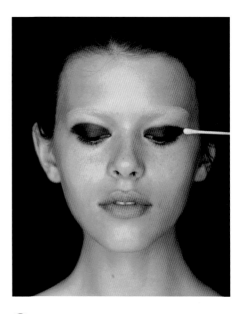

2 DEFINITION

Using a black kohl pencil, heavily line under each eye and blacken the outer edges of each lid, then smudge the edges of the pencil into the blue pigment.

3 BLENDING

Looking up, blend the same blue pigment you used on your eyelids on top of the kohl pencil on your lower lash lines. You can clean up any fallout later.

Because the model's eyebrows were bleached on a previous shoot, they're looking a bit yellow, so I applied a creamy foundation to a clean mascara wand and combed it through.

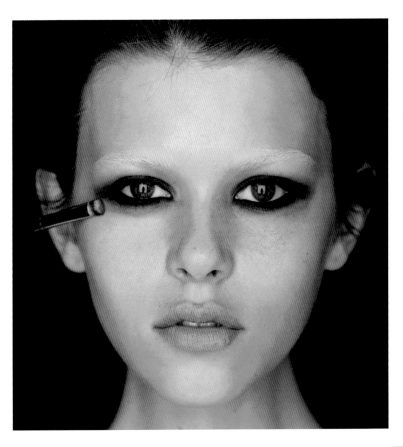

4 EYE SHADOW & BLENDING

Blend a lavender eye shadow around your whole eye until any hard edges disappear. Repeat for the other eye.

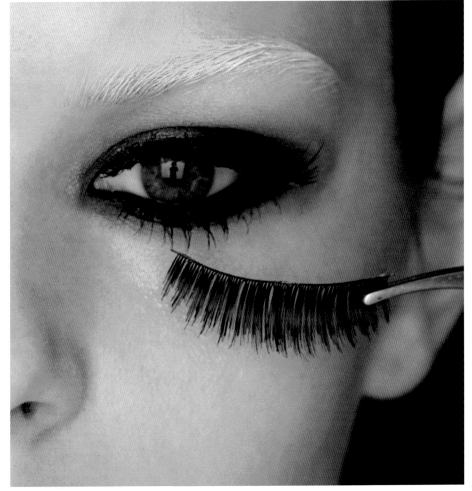

5 LASHES, CHEEKS & LIPS

Clean up any fallout, curl your lashes and apply as much mascara as humanly possible. Apply false full lashes, as shown. Use liquid foundation, then finish off with a soft, nude coral lipstick. Rub the same lipstick onto your fingertips and pat it onto your cheeks as a blush.

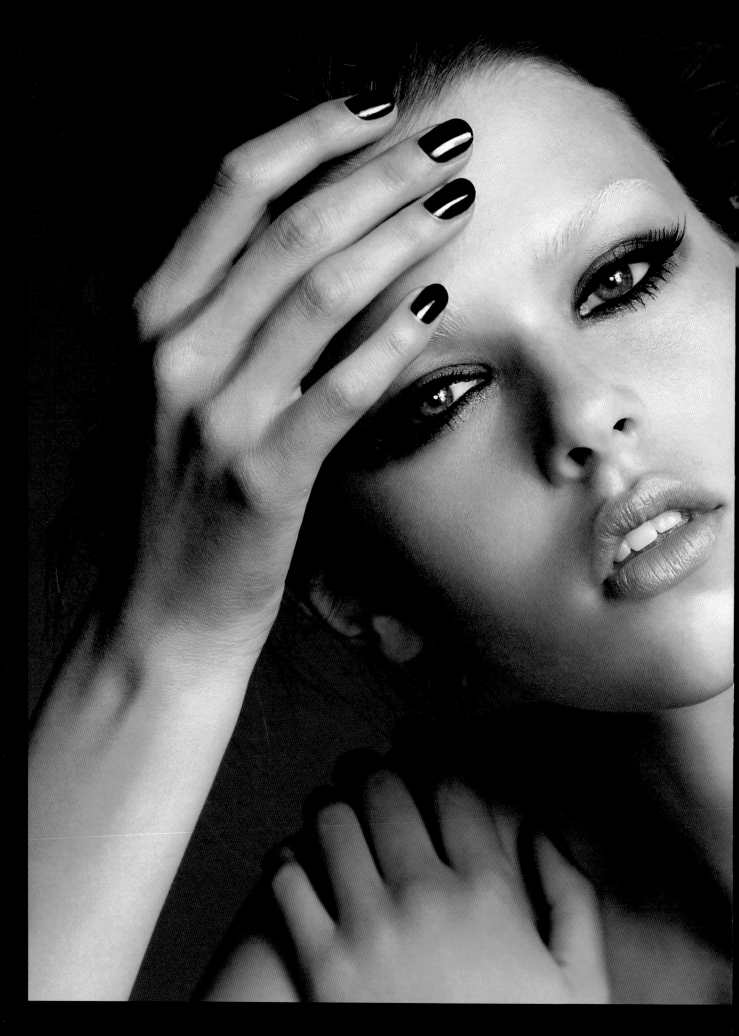

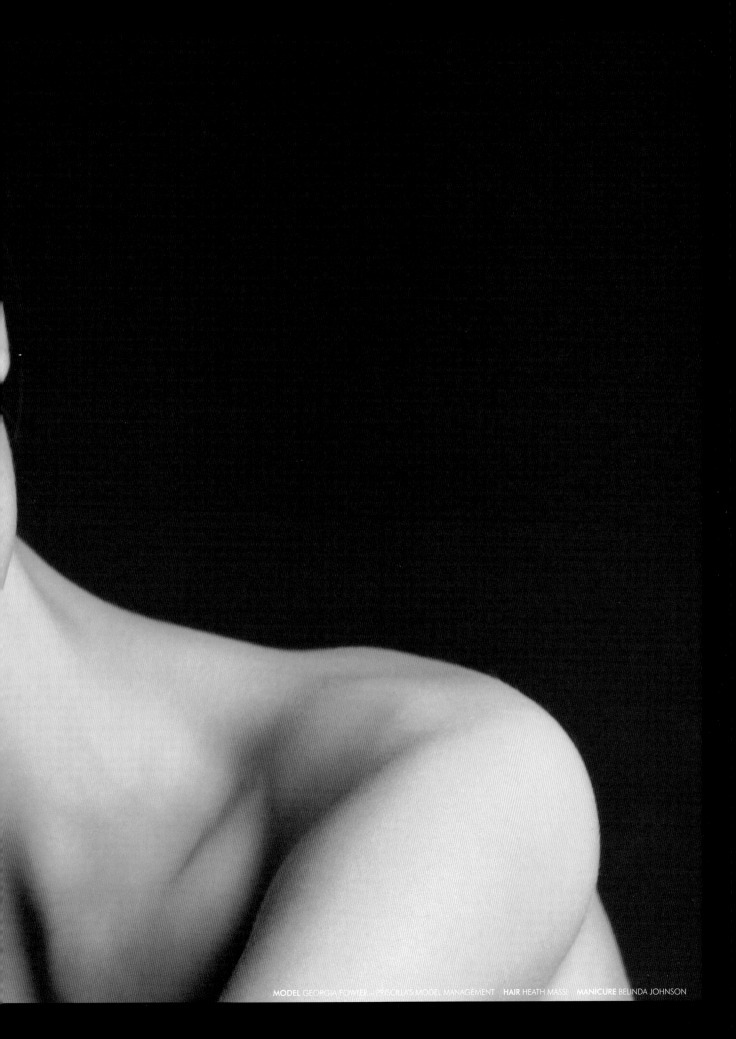

30 | ROCK STARLET

A PALE CREAMY LOOK
THAT'S PERFECT FOR
TAWNY BLONDES.

1 PREP, BROWS & LASHES

Prep your skin, then
apply liquid foundation
and concealer. Powder
all over, including your
eyelids. I've lightened
Natalie's brows with
brow mascara, then
applied a creamy white
pencil to her inner rims.
Curl your lashes and apply
lots of mascara to your
top and bottom lashes.

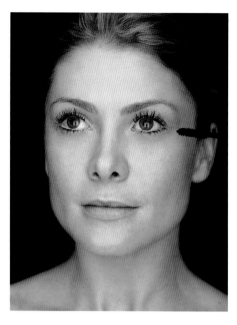

2 EYE SHADOW & BROWS

Apply a soft wash of
taupe eye shadow under
your eyes and over your
entire eyelids, then blend
the edges with a light
translucent powder.
Define your brows.

3 BRONZER & HIGHLIGHTER

Add a soft bronzer—more
of a caramel tone than
an orange one—to your
cheeks. Highlight your
lips and the inner corners
of your eyes. A soft nude
lip works well with this
look. If you have an extra
five minutes, apply some
single lashes.

*If you're blond and want to
lighten your brow but don't
have a brow mascara, put a little
foundation on a clean mascara
wand and comb it through.*

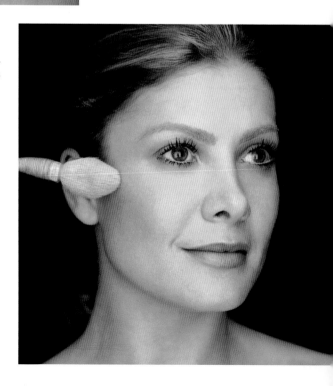

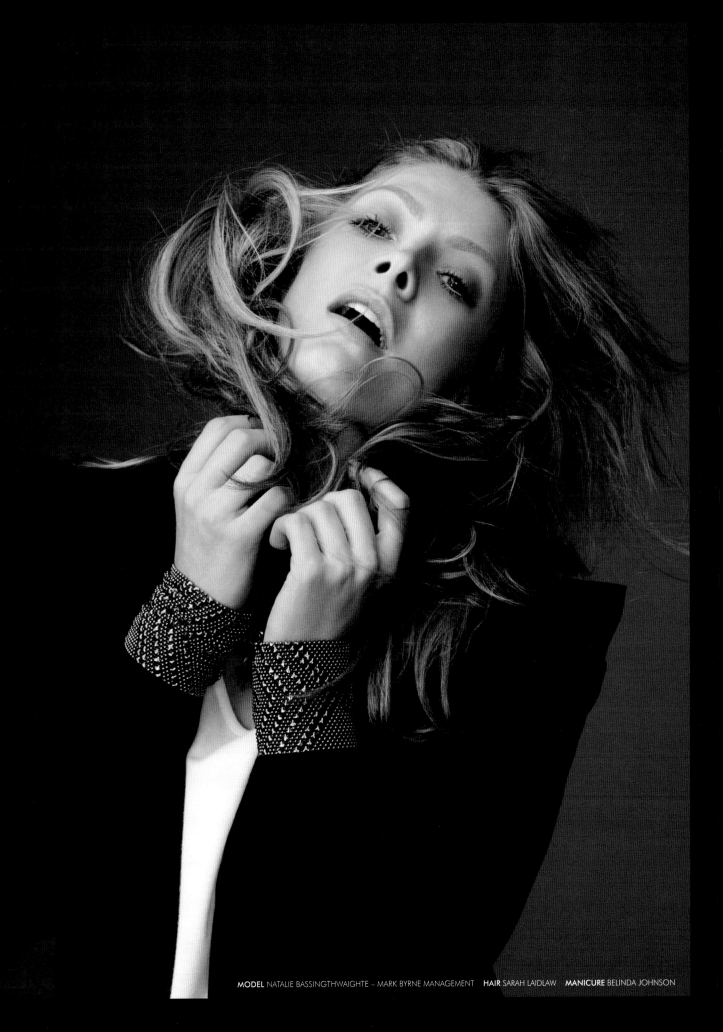

MODEL NATALIE BASSINGTHWAIGHTE – MARK BYRNE MANAGEMENT   HAIR SARAH LAIDLAW   MANICURE BELINDA JOHNSON

31 | FEMME FATALE

HOLLYWOOD GLAMOUR
FOR DRAMA QUEENS.

1 PREP, PIGMENT & EYE SHADOW

Prep your skin and apply cream foundation. Add a soft wash of gold pigment to your eyelids, then a matte taupe eye shadow just under your brow bones. Highlight the inner corners with a silver pigment.

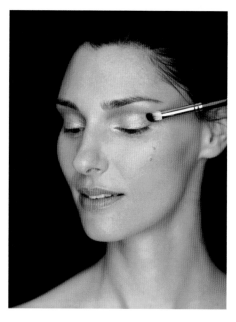

2 EYELINER & LASHES

Use an angle brush to lightly smudge black gel eyeliner along your top lash lines. Curl your lashes, and apply lots of black mascara to your top lashes only. Apply false 3/4 lashes. In this shot I've already applied the lashes and I'm holding up another one so you can see the lash type.

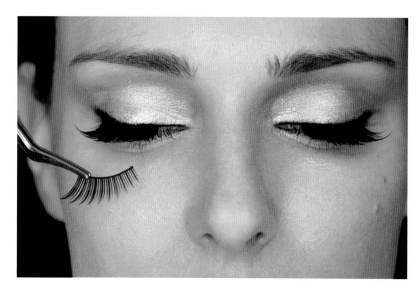

3 POWDER, CHEEKS & LIPS

Powder your whole face with translucent powder, then apply a creamy white pencil to the lower inner rim of each eye. Apply a dark burgundy lipstick, then a very soft rose-coloured blush to your cheeks. With a dark nail polish, this is a strong look that makes a statement.

Only use the silver pigment if it suits your eye colour; otherwise, just stick to the gold.

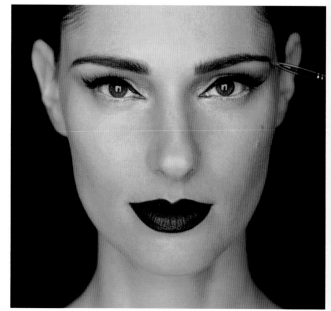

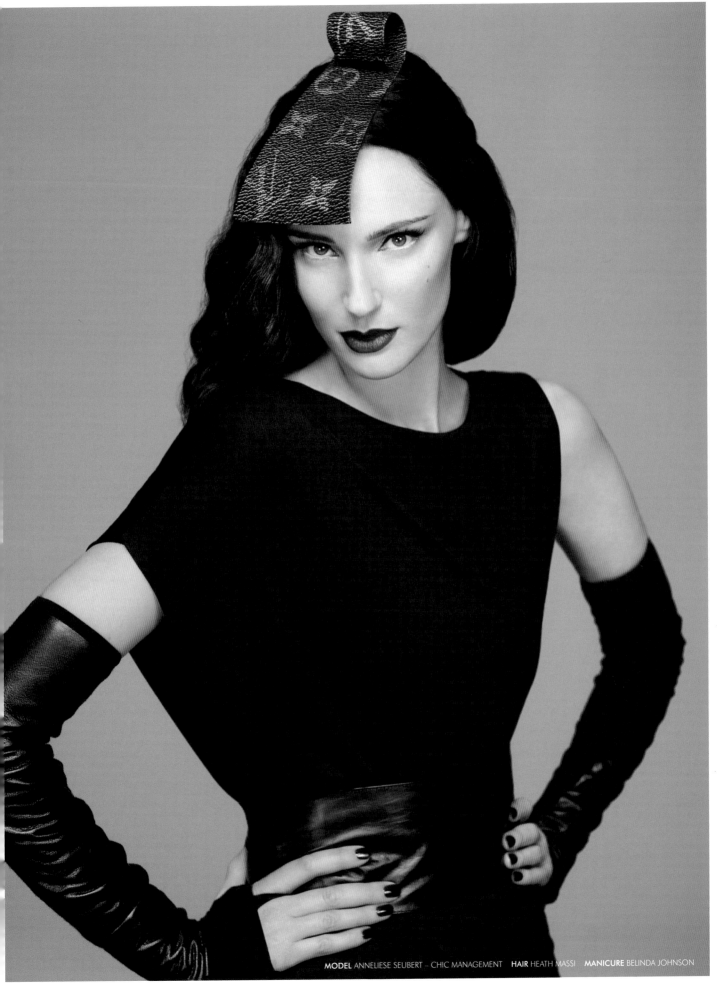

32 | FRESCO CHIC

VOLUPTUOUS NATURAL
LIPS, THE PERFECT FOIL
FOR A STRONG EYE.

1 PREP & LASHES

Prep your skin, then
apply foundation and
concealer. Apply powder
all over, especially
your eyelids. This gives
a velvety finish. Curl
your lashes and apply
mascara, then apply
false 3/4 lashes to your
top lashes only.

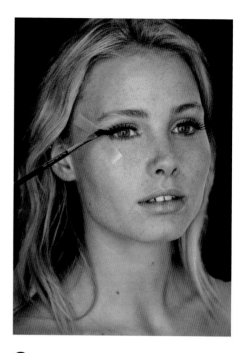

2 EYELINER

Use sticky tape as a stencil,
but stick it to an item of
clothing a few times so it
loses some of its adhesive.
Imagine a line running from
the corner of your nose to
the outside of your eye.
This is the angle at which
to apply the sticky tape.
Trust me, this will lift your
eye. Make sure you apply
the eyeliner while looking
straight into the mirror. Use
a black eye shadow, rather
than a liquid, because liquids
can crack and look harsh
(cream eyeliners are also
a fantastic option).

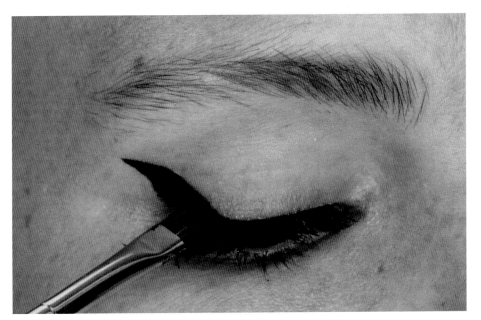

3 EYELINER

When you look down a little, you'll notice a gap in the eyeliner. That's because you've done the eyeliner looking straight ahead. Fill in the little gap, then continue your liner along your top lash line towards the inner corner of your eye. Repeat for the other eye. Now when you're looking straight ahead, you'll have a perfect eyeliner that lifts your eyes.

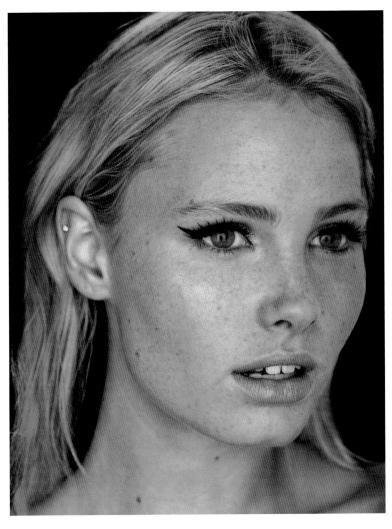

4 CHEEKS, LIPS & LASHES

Contour your cheeks with matte brown eye shadow, but don't apply coloured blush to your cheeks. This darkens under your cheekbones; see the full step-by-step in *Makeup: The Ultimate Guide* (2008), pages 162–7. Matte down your lips with a nude lipstick so they will look fuller and more voluptuous. Lipsticks have more pigment than lip glosses, so they can knock out natural lip colour, whereas sheer glosses aren't always strong enough. To finish this look, apply lots of mascara to your bottom lashes.

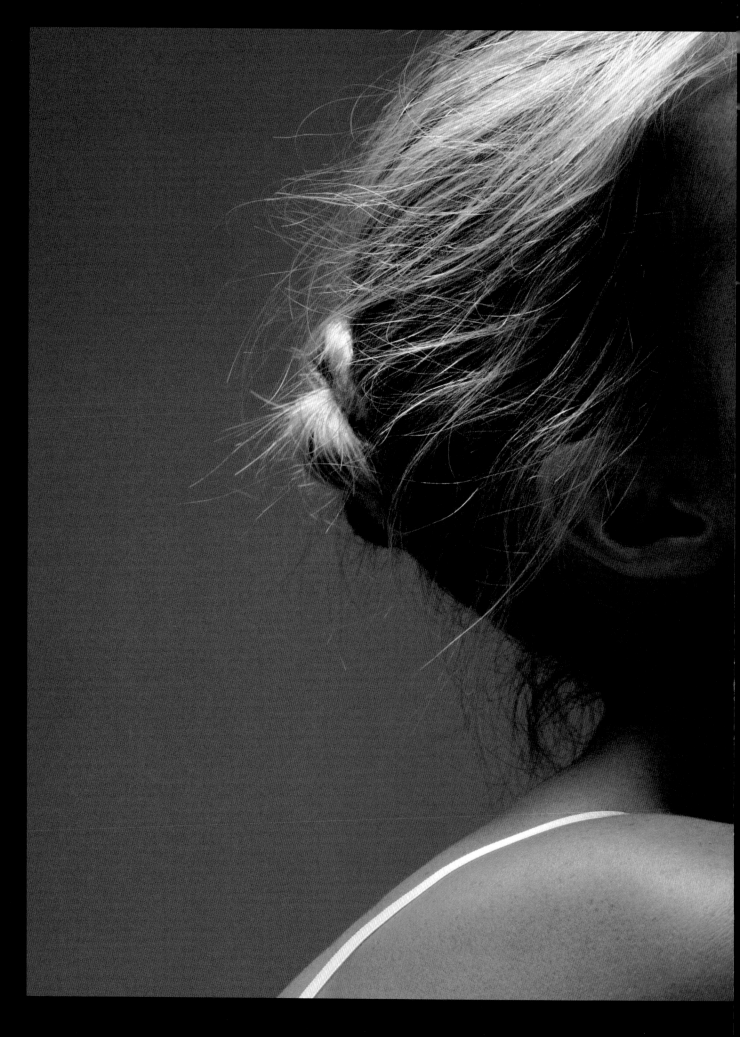

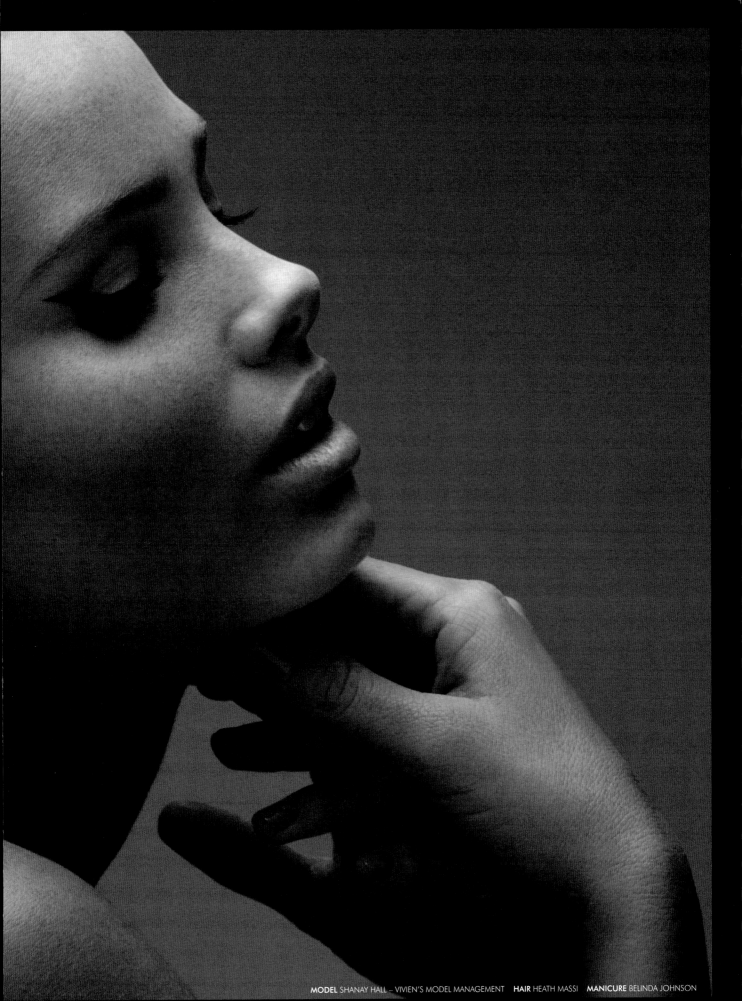

33 | MIDNIGHT METALS

SHIMMER AT NIGHT WITH
THIS INTENSE GLITTER EYE.

1 CREAM & LASH GLUE

When creating an intense glitter eye, you must be careful—first, read the instructions on page 114. Apply cream under your eyes and latex all over your eyelids, then wait a couple of seconds for the eyelash glue to become tacky.

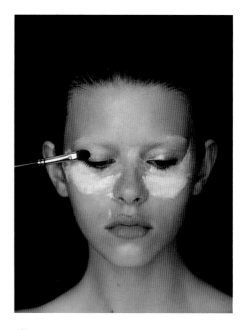

2 GLITTER

Latex is impossible to remove from brushes so, when applying glitter to the latex, use a brush you can afford to ruin. Apply all over your lids, up to your brows.

3 HIGHLIGHTING GLITTER

Looking down, apply a bit of extra latex to the centre of each eyelid. Add glitter in a lighter colour to this area to make it stand out. With your eyes shut, use the hairdryer to blow any excess away, then clean up all the fallout. Use double-sided sticky tape to remove any excess glitter that has fallen onto your cheeks.

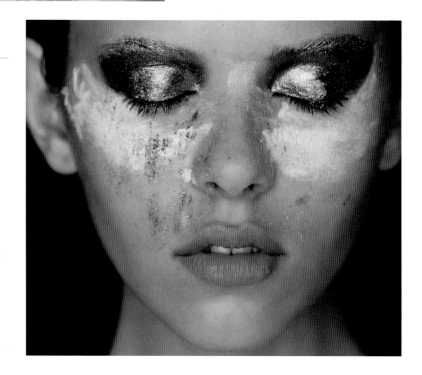

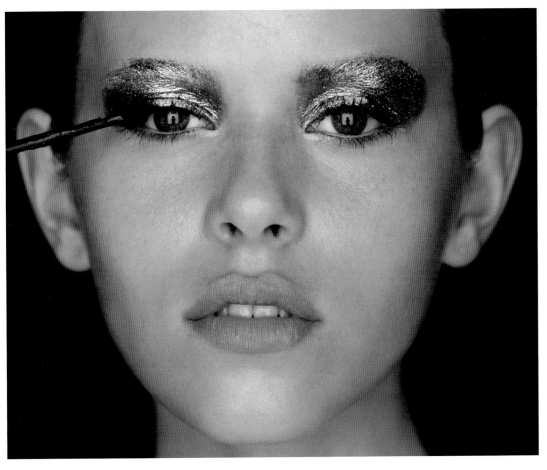

4 LOWER DEFINITION & LASHES

Using a pale blue pencil, line your lower inner eye rims. Then curl your lashes, and apply heavy mascara to your top lashes only.

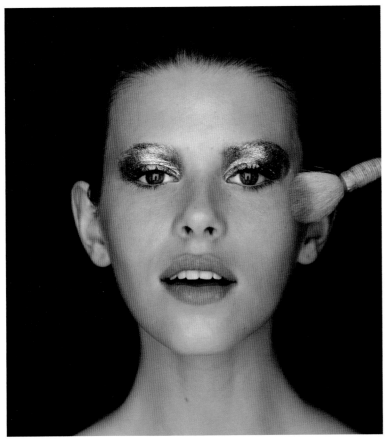

5 CHEEKS & LIPS

Finish off with a soft berry cream blush and a natural lip balm. If you have pale lips, pop a hint of cream blush on your lips, or mix it with the lip balm.

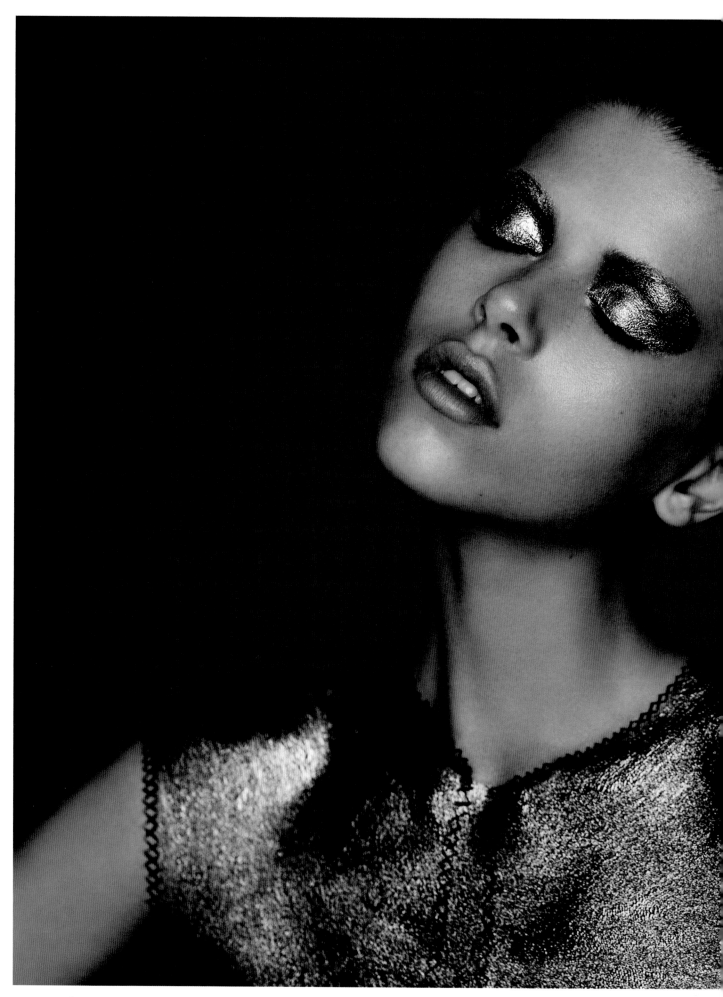

34 | MOD GLOSS

A STRONGLY DEFINED EYE
WITH A FLASH OF SILVER.

1 EYE PREP, KOHL & LASHES

If your skin is clear, prep your eyes only. Line the inner rim of your eye and the end of the bottom lash line with a metallic silver kohl pencil. Repeat for the other eye. Curl your lashes and apply lots of mascara to your top and bottom lashes.

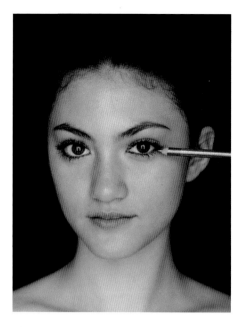

2 EYELINER & BLENDING

Keeping the shape quite square, apply black liquid eyeliner straight across your top lids. Wait for it to dry, then take the same eyeliner along the bottom eyelash line, flicking it out along the edge. Use a sharp angle brush for precision.

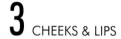

3 CHEEKS & LIPS

Apply a rosy pink cream blush and a nude matte lipstick. You can use a lip pencil as lipstick here, but make sure you colour in your whole lip.

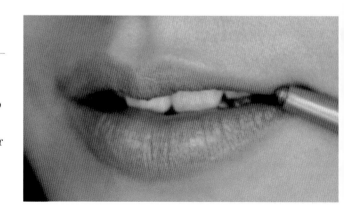

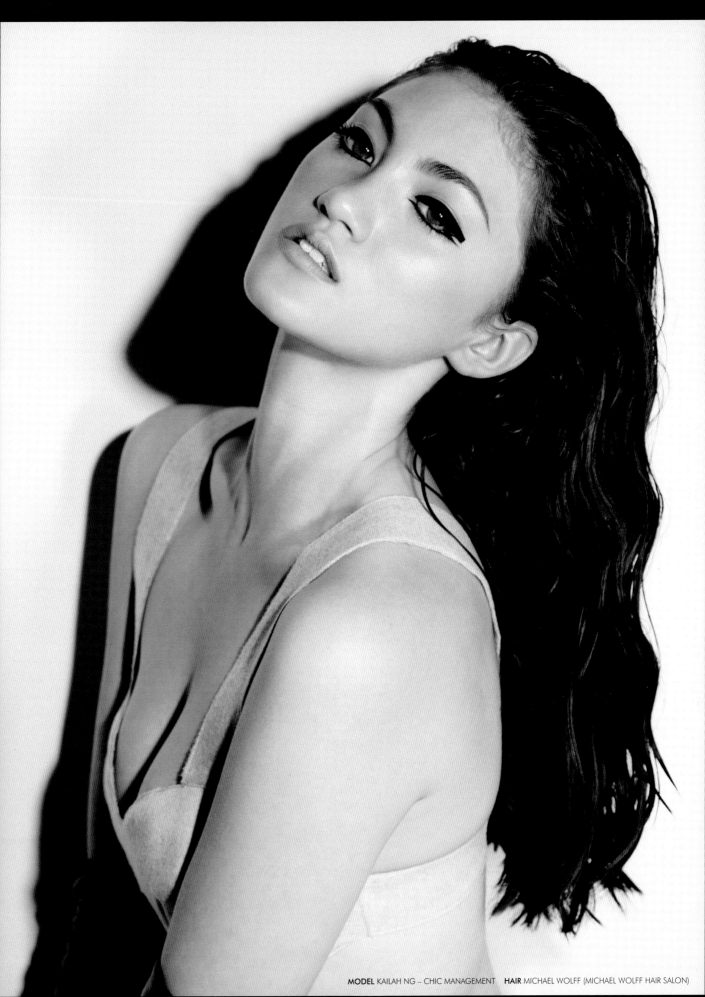

35 ETERNAL SUMMER

LOTS OF GIRLS CRAVE
THE 'WET LOOK', SO
HERE'S HOW IT'S DONE.

1 PREP, EYE SHADOW & HIGHLIGHTER

This look doesn't last, so keep a mirror handy for constant checks. Apply foundation, and concealer if necessary. Don't powder your eyelids. Apply cream eye shadow to your eyelids and blend it up to your eyebrows. It will give you a shiny 'wet' effect. Alternatively, use gold shimmer eye shadow.

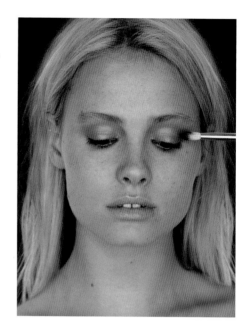

2 DEFINITION

Highlight your skin. Apply a soft wash of gold eye shadow under your eyelids, then define your lash lines with a chocolate-brown pencil and blend together.

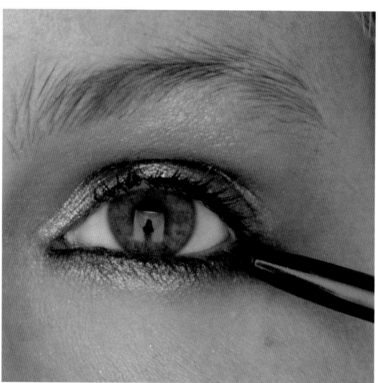

Cream eye shadows are rare and hard to find. Sometimes I create my own by mixing eye shadow with lip balm!

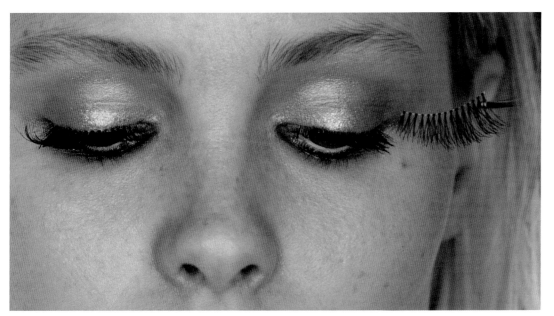

3 LASHES & BROWS

Curl your lashes, then apply lots of black mascara to your top lashes. I've applied false wispy lashes to give each eye a winged effect. Apply a creamy white pencil to the inner rims of your eyes to open and refresh them. Then define your brows with a pencil that matches your brow colour.

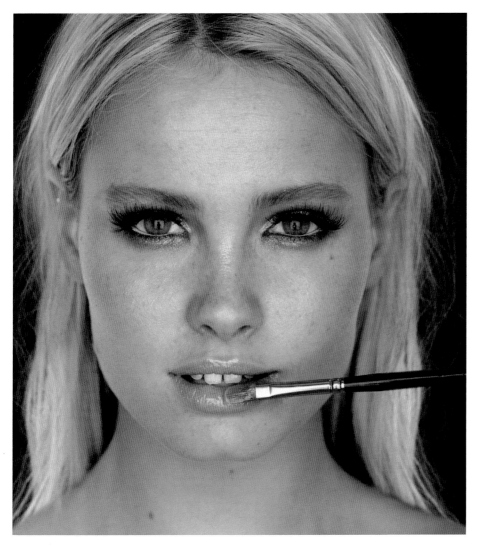

4 CHEEKS & LIPS

Apply lots of golden cream bronzer to your cheeks and blend well with a kabuki brush, then highlight your cheekbones with a gold cream highlighter. Finish off with a tangerine lip gloss.

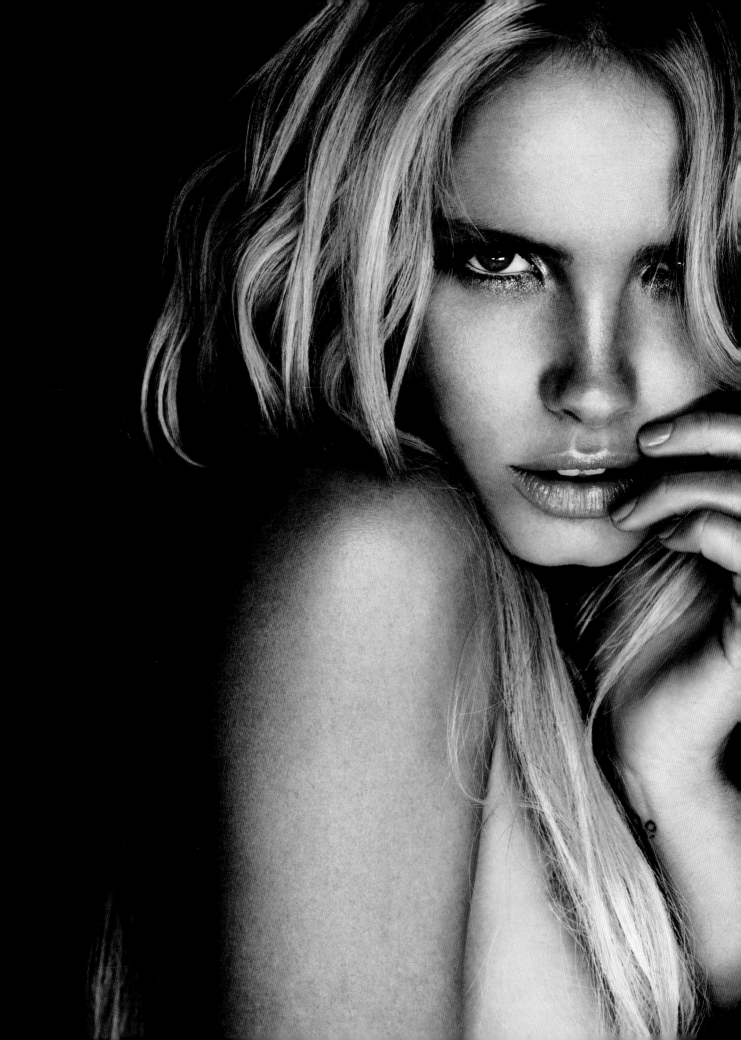

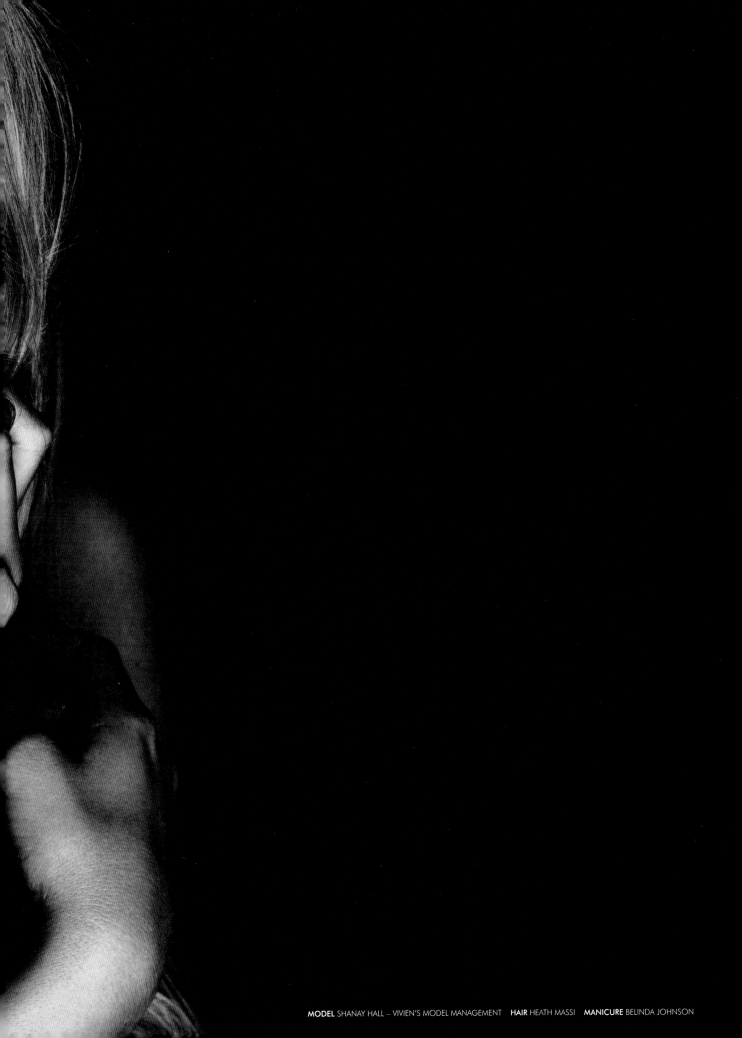

36 | ORCHID SMILE

A FRESH GLAMOROUS
LOOK WITH SWISH
SHIMMERY HIGHLIGHTS.

1 PREP, POWDER & CHEEKS

Apply foundation, and
concealer where required.
Powder all over, then
apply a bright tangerine
orange blush to your
cheeks. The model has
fabulous skin, so I've used
a shimmery blush, but if
you're conscious of fine
lines around your eyes,
keep the blush matte.

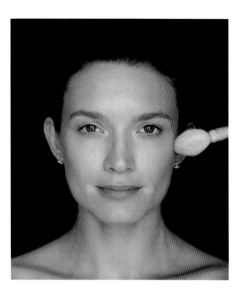

2 DEFINITION

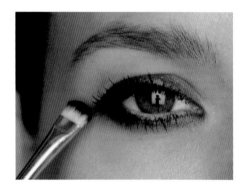

Take a chocolate-brown eye pencil and
smudge it around your whole eye. Don't
worry if it looks a little rough—it just
needs to heat up on your skin for a minute
so it becomes easier to smudge. Repeat for
the other eye.

3 LASHES

Use a mini square blending brush to
smudge that pencil and extend the
edges. Curl your lashes and apply lots of
mascara to your top and bottom lashes.

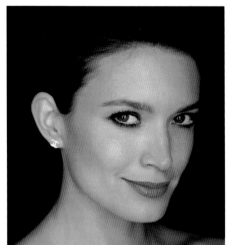

4 LIPS & BROWS

Finish off with a bright
orange matte lipstick.
Wet your brush, then
add shimmery gold
pigment to the inner
corners of your eyes.
Finally, lightly define
your brows.

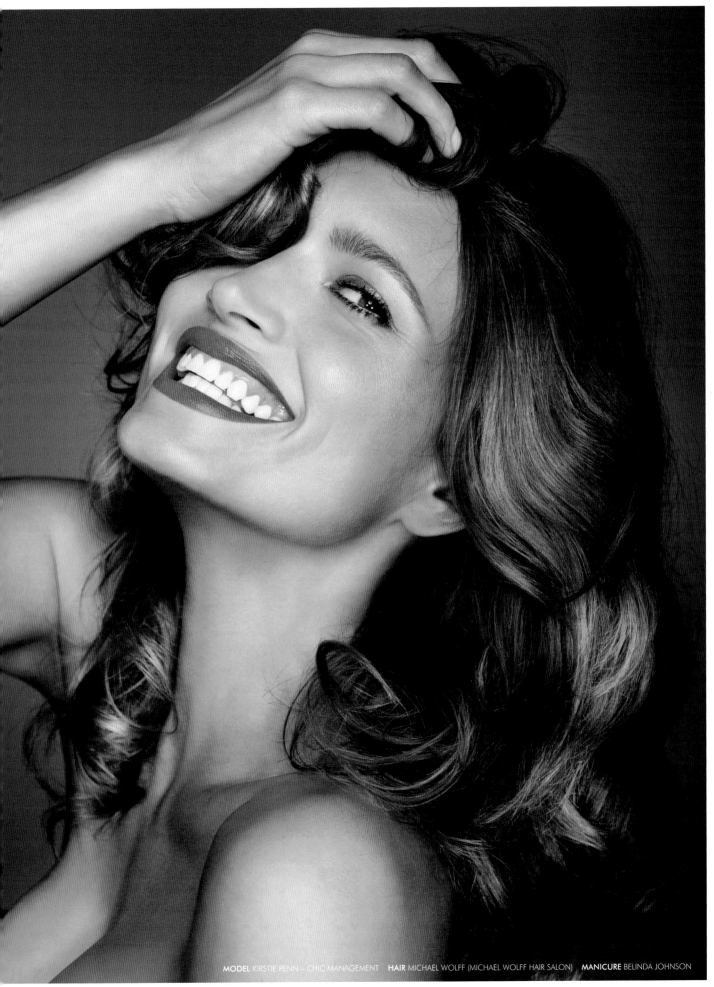

37 EXQUISITE DEFINITION

SUMMON YOUR INNER
ROCK CHICK WITH SMOKY
EYES AND NUDE LIPS.

1 EYE PREP

Because this look
requires soft, smoky
eyes, just apply sheer
liquid foundation,
then lightly powder
your eyelids so that
you can blend perfectly.

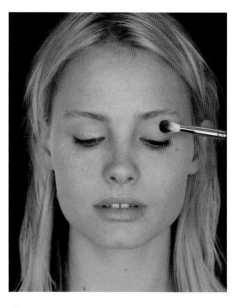

2 EYE SHADOW

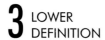

With a medium eye shadow brush,
apply a soft, matte grey eye shadow
along your entire eyelids, stopping
under your brow bones. If you have
trouble blending your eye shadow,
pick up translucent powder with a
clean brush and use it to blend.

3 LOWER DEFINITION

Use a medium-sized brush
to apply the same colour
under your eyes, then use
an angle brush to apply
a darker shade of grey
along the lash line.

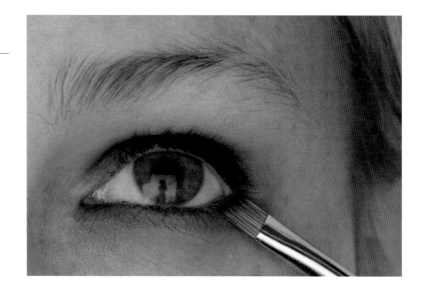

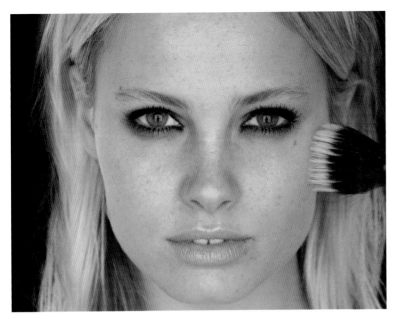

4 EYES, LASHES & HIGHLIGHTER

Apply a black kohl pencil along your top and bottom lash lines, then softly smudge with a small eye shadow brush. Curl your lashes, apply lots of black mascara to your top and bottom lashes and clean up any fallout. Use sheer liquid foundation mixed with luminiser to highlight your skin all over.

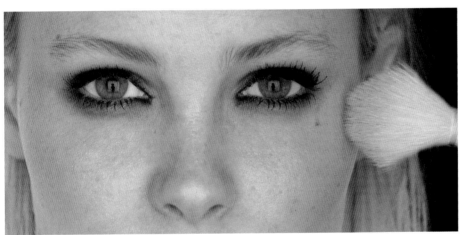

5 CHEEKS

Conceal any blemishes. Using a kabuki brush, apply cream blush high on your cheeks. Don't smile as you apply blush, or you'll create lines.

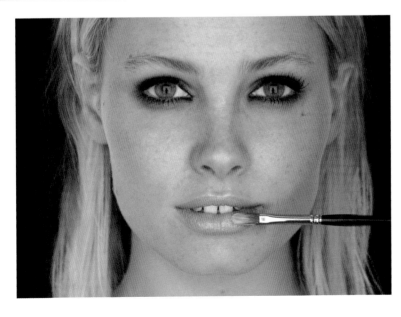

6 LIPS

This look is great with just a little bit of lip balm, but you can even out your lips with a nude lipstick.

MODEL SHANAY HALL – VIVIEN'S MODEL MANAGEMENT   HAIR HEATH MASSI

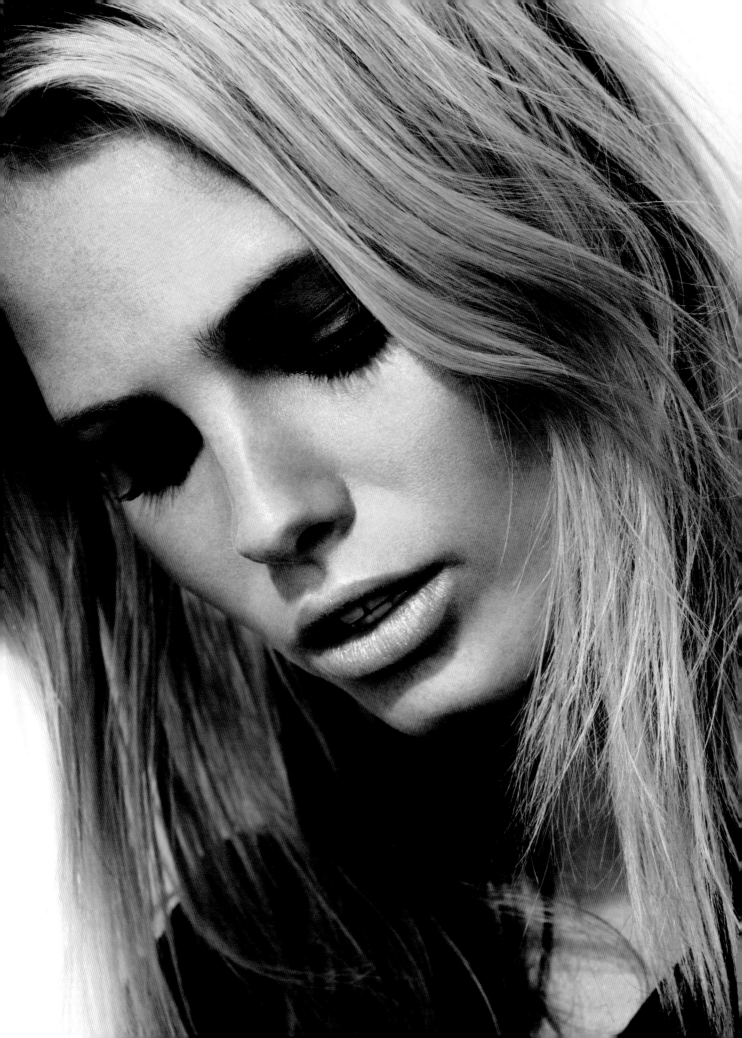

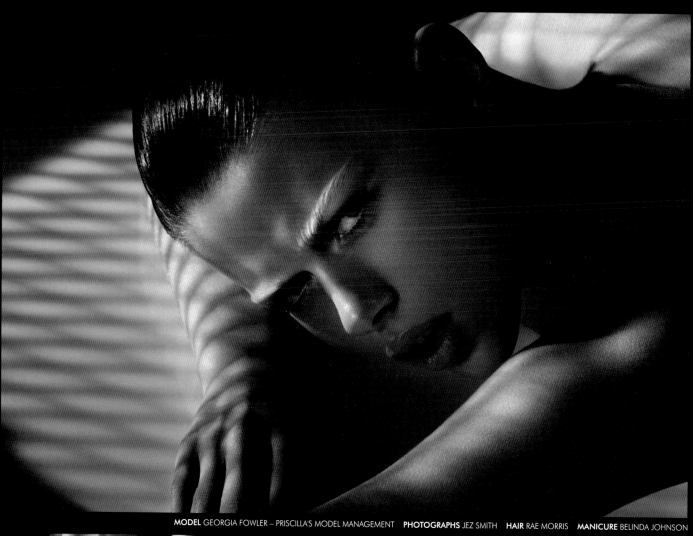

MODEL GEORGIA FOWLER – PRISCILLA'S MODEL MANAGEMENT   **PHOTOGRAPHS** JEZ SMITH   **HAIR** RAE MORRIS   **MANICURE** BELINDA JOHNSON

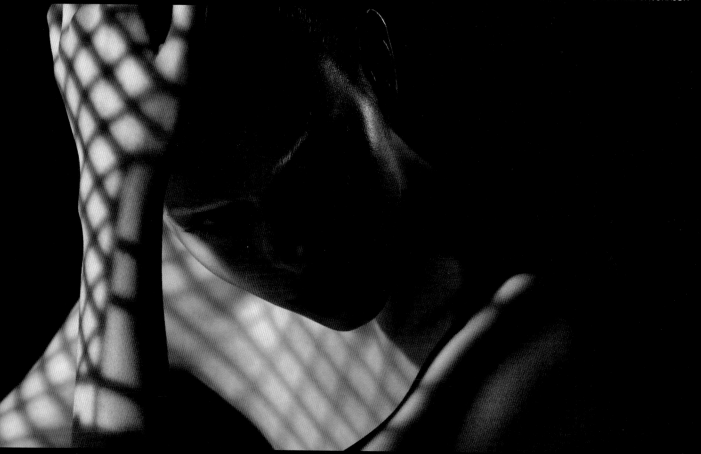

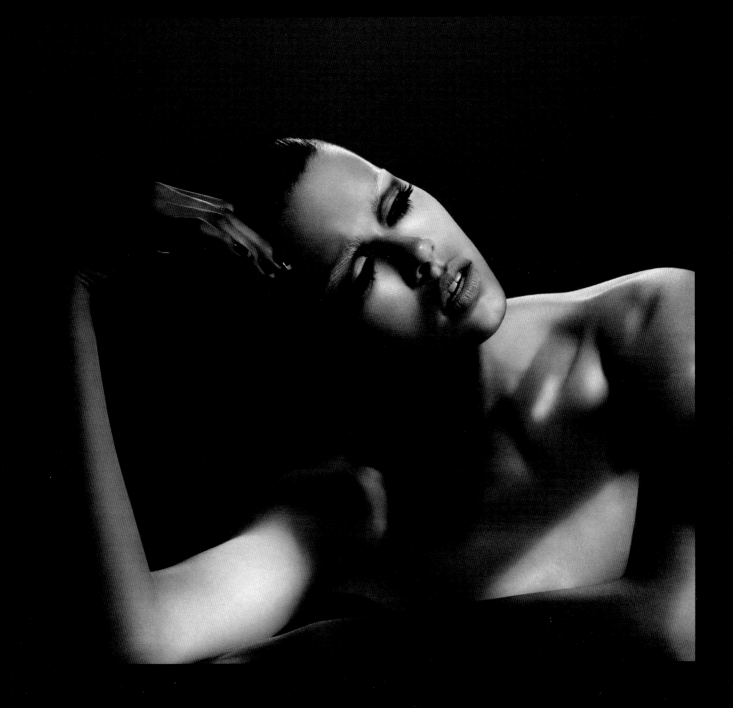

www.RAEMORRIS.com

Index

Acknowledgments

Two makeup masters—Richard Dechazel and my mentor, Richard Sharah—taught me most of what I know and are responsible for where I am today.

Richard Dechazel allowed me to assist him and helped me become a better makeup artist. He's a genius. I've long since forgiven his temper tantrums, screaming, yelling, and also the occasional flying makeup brushes I had to duck! Richard, I thank you.

As for Richard Sharah—well, tears just well up when I think of him. He passed away not so long ago. Many of the world's makeup artists will agree that he was the god of makeup. And yet the man who designed the Ziggy Stardust makeup for David Bowie, and was famous for creating the models' look in the Robert Palmer film clip 'Simply Irresistible', was colour blind. Can you believe it? I feel incredibly lucky to have been Richard's last student. To do this day, I still hear his voice in my head saying 'Blend, Rae, blend.'

And to my fellow up-and-coming makeup artists, look up Richard Sharah on the internet. Be prepared to be yelled at, broke, tired and even a 'starving artist'. To reach the top as a makeup artist, you have to immerse yourself 24/7 with makeup, fashion magazines and inspirational websites. Knowledge is power. You must be at the forefront of trends, constantly looking at international shows, knowing which makeup artist directs what, which photographers are shooting what, and who the 'It' girls are. I also believe that makeup has to be 'in your blood'. If you're meant to be a makeup artist, you'll do all the things I've outlined above without hesitating.

Finally, a huge thank you to all the people who've made this book possible.

Steven Chee – photographer; Geoffrey Burger Nolan – stylist; Benjamin Croft – designer and art director; Grace Testa (www.gracetesta.com) – retoucher; and Bronwyn Fraser (www.styleestablishment.com.au) – colour expert.

My literary agents Mark Byrne and Lisa Hanrahan; my publisher Louise Thurtell and editor Alexandra Nahlous; project manager Sarah Baker; and the incredible Kate Hyde.

Tobias Rowles – digital operator; Duncan Pickett – photographic assistant; Lei Tai – my right-hand makeup assistant; Kathy Criniti – makeup assistant; Casey Gore – makeup assistant; Gina Guirguis – makeup assistant; Michael Shiailis – makeup assistant; Elena Gomez – typist/text formatter; Phaedra Giblin – typist/makeup assistant; and Katherine Teroxy – Geoffrey Burger Nolan's assistant.

Heath Massi – hair stylist; Sarah Laidlaw – hair stylist; Michael Wolff (Michael Wolff Hair Salon) – hair stylist; Joel Phillips – hair stylist; Belinda Johnson – manicurist (www.belbeautyandnails.com); and Cameron Jane, Samantha Robinson and Flor Sepulveda – Cameron Jane Makeup School.

Ursula Hufnagl and Yonta Taiwo at Chic Management; and all the fabulous models at Chic Management – Cassi Colvin, Erika Heynatz, Miranda Kerr, Catherine McNeil, Shadae Magson, Kailah Ng, Kirstie Penn, Anneliese Seubert, Sarah Stephens and Kieta Van Ewyk.

Jaz Daly at Priscilla's Model Management; and models at Priscilla's Model Management – Kate Alstegren, Chrystal Copland, Alice Dickman, Kerry Doyle, Georgia Fowler, Ruby Grose, Tess Haubrich, Caitlin Lomax, Eve Lui, Tina Malou and Cornelia Tat.

Susie Deveridge and Tineke Dickson at Vivien's Model Management; and models at Vivien's Model Management – Kuei Alor, Lauren Beasley, Brigette Burk, Jenny Day, Rachael Grasso, Shanay Hall, Millicent Lambor and Lynn Sutherland.

Sarah Grant at Chadwick Models; and model at Chadwick Models – Samantha Basalari.

Ruby Rose and Natalie Bassingthwaighte – Mark Byrne Management.

Rosie Tupper – Viva London (London) and DNA (New York).

Wendy Tomaino – Smiink Eyelashes and Ultimate Brush Roll.

Jez Smith for the photograph of Rae Morris on the black flap.

DLM; Luxe Studios; The Front for supplying extra lights and equipment; Juliet Fallowfield and Amelia – Chanel; Kenneth Beck – www.carbon8.com.au.

Fashion credits

iv and **129** Bodysuit: This is Genevieve; Arm bands: Suzy O'Rourke.
vi, **viii** and **158–9** Clothes: Christopher Esber.
2–3 Props and accessories: Stylist's own.
20 Ring and scarf: Vintage.
22–3 Mini turban headband: Stylist's own.
26–7 Bra: Stylist's own; Jewellery: Kerry Rocks.

40–1, 58–9, 66–7 and **76–7** Bra and gloves: Stylist's own; Sheer top: Tim O'Connor; Jewellery: Kerry Rocks.

46–7 Bra and gloves: Stylist's own; Sheer top and faux fur jacket: Tim O'Connor; Jewellery: Kerry Rocks.

75 Necklace: Christian Dior.

82–3 Tank top: Nathan Smith; White boy pants: Holeproof; Necklace: Christian Dior.

85 Tank top: Nathan Smith.

87 Tank top: Nathan Smith.

90–1 Necklace, black bracelet and round ring: Chanel; Small ring, round bracelets and earrings: Peep Toe.

93 Necklace: Chanel; Top: Nathan Smith.

95 White dress shirt: Nathan Smith.

101 Top and skirt: Sara Phillips.

103 All-in-one: Billion Dollar Babes; Hat: Suzy O'Rourke; Rubber gloves: Reactor; Bag: Stylist's own.

105 White shirt: Sara Phillips; Hat: Suzy O'Rourke.

107 Tank top: Nathan Smith; Earrings: Kate McCoy.

109 Dress and top: Alistair Trung.

111 Black button shirt: Christopher Esber; Black skull cap: Suzy O'Rourke; Gloves: Alistair Trung; Bowtie: World.

113 Earrings: Stylist's own.

115 Headpiece: Suzy O'Rourke; Flowered jumpsuit: Billion Dollar Babes.

121 Bodysuit: Evil Twin; Jacket: Jack London; Bracelets: Diva.

126–7 All clothing: Chanel.

132–3 White shirt: Alistair Trung.

136–7 Jacket: Tim O'Connor; Shoulder adornment: Headband by Diva.

139 Dress: Mink Pink; Headpiece: Suzy O'Rourke.

141 Jacket (beige): Sara Phillips; Jacket (black): Christopher Esber; Studded denim shorts: One Teaspoon; Earrings: Stylist's own.

146–7 All jewellery: Christian Dior; Gloves: Master and Slave; Skirt: Toni Maticevski; Metal bra: Christopher Esber.

153 White top: Mink Pink; Necklaces: Christian Dior; Cuffs: Diva; Jacket: Manning Cartell.

155 Dress: Christopher Esber; Belt and gauntlets: Alistair Trung; Paper accessory concept: Geoffrey Burger Nolan.

162–3 T-shirt concept: Rae Morris.

165 Bra top: Stylist's own; Gloves: Alistair Trung.

168–9 One-shoulder dress: Christopher Esber.

174–5 Clothes: Christopher Esber.

First published in 2010

Arena Books, an imprint of
Allen & Unwin
83 Alexander Street
Crows Nest NSW 2065
Australia
Phone: (61 2) 8425 0100
Fax: (61 2) 9906 2218
Email: info@allenandunwin.com
Web: www.allenandunwin.com

Cataloguing-in-Publication details are available from
the National Library of Australia
www.librariesaustralia.nla.gov.au

ISBN 978 1 74237 339 3

Design by Benjamin Croft
Printed in China at Everbest Printing Co
10 9 8 7 6 5 4